# COPE WITH IT!

# DR. LAURA SCHLESSINGER

# COPE WITH IT!

KENSINGTON BOOKS
*http://www.kensingtonbooks.com*

KENSINGTON BOOKS are published by

Kensington Publishing Corp.
850 Third Avenue
New York, NY 10022

All Kensington titles, imprints and distributed lines are available at special quantity discounts for bulk purchases for sales promotion, premiums, fund raising, educational or institutional use.

Special book excerpts or customized printings can also be created to fit specific needs. For details, write or phone the office of the Kensington Special Sales Manager: Kensington Publishing Corp., 850 Third Avenue, New York, NY, Attn. Special Sales Department. Phone: 1-800-221-2647.

ISBN 1-57566-855-6

First Kensington Printing: September, 2000
10 9 8 7 6 5 4 3 2 1

Printed in the United States of America

# Contents

# CHAPTER 1

# Parents, Children, Family

Do you get all upset when your parents offer an opinion? When you were a kid and your parents said, "Now, dear, I don't think that's a good idea," you probably took those words to heart. Maybe in your family, advice was really a threat or an order, but even if it wasn't, all children are inexperienced and insecure and look to parents for direction and applause. What better way to walk the straight and narrow than to follow your parents' advice? Now you're all grown up. You complain about your parents' interference. You fight them. You ignore them. It's possible that your parents are not making demands. It's possible that you are still insecure and needy of applause from your mom and dad, and when either one disagrees with you, it highlights your insecurity. The real danger is your own emotional wobbliness and not your parents' demands. If you hear their expression of feelings and opinions as demands, you're still the little kid you used to be.

When your kid fails, do you feel let down? In the movie *The Bad News Bears,* the father of one of the Little League ballplayers became enraged whenever his son's pitch put a player on base. The father verbally and physically abused his son in front of everyone. With the bases loaded, his son pitched, and the batter bunted. The boy caught the ball and held on to it until all four opponents scored. This little boy discovered that the way to fight his father was to allow himself to fail. Is that what you force your children into? Must your children become failures as their only way to establish an identity separate from your ego? Your child is not an extension of you. Your child is a separate human being. It's not your child's responsibility to justify your existence, but to explore life, to build and enjoy his own existence. Help your child to maximize himself. Don't own his successes. Applaud them.

Just you wait till Daddy gets home! That vigil for Father's return from work is a nightmare for your child, a frustration for you, and a sad welcome for Dad. Mom, that phrase makes Dad the family hit man and you the family snitch, both unsavory positions in gangster movies and families. That phrase is also a testament to your feelings of helplessness in relating to your children. It's easy for kids to drive you into feeling that way. They test, push, question, whine, attack, threaten, and use any other tactic they can dream up. It's not a rational Waltons family exchange all the time. To function and survive as a mother, you need two basics: an independent sense of value and a loyal, loving contract with their dad that says it's you and him against them. The independent sense of value will give you the strength to stand your ground, use your imagination, and not feel annihilated by failure or their disobedience. That loving contract with Dad eliminates your kids' access to playing you off each other. It makes you someone to contend with.

How can you keep your kids away from other kids you don't like because they're probably a bad influence? If your child has one or a few friends you feel are undesirable, I suggest you hold back on coming all unglued and laying down impossible rules. If you get carried away enough, you might become the most undesirable creature in your child's life. The first thing you need to do is look at your child carefully and honestly. Please don't mix up different with bad. Outside of superficial things like hair and dress styles, is your kid basically a good kid, a nice person? If the answer is no, then I would suggest family therapy. But if your answer is yes, then I would suggest your being clever. If your child sees something in someone, trust your child, and respect what they see. You can talk about your reservations only if you're willing to listen to your child's explanations. Show interest in this undesirable child. You may learn something. At the very least, your child won't be made to feel that acceptance and understanding have to be sought outside the home.

Do you wish your family would get off your back? You have work to do. You have responsibilities, deadlines, obligations. There isn't enough time for you to take care of them at work, so of course, you have to do them at home. Whether it's calculations on paper or worry on your mind, your kids, your spouse, your dog, your neighbors, your friends just don't seem to understand this. They nag, complain, grab at you, demand time, get in your way. You resent them—tinged with some guilt that, well, you should be giving them their time also. My question for you is this: When is it your turn to get? Think about it. You're feeling all spent out. You gave at the office. You feel like you've got to give more at home. When is it your turn to get? You've probably asked yourself that question already, annoyed that no one is giving to you. But your notion of your family giving to you is leaving you alone. Brace yourself. You aren't getting because you aren't allowing it. You're so involved in winning and doing, you deny yourself and you push your loved ones away. Is playing with your kids really all for *them*?

Are you being too good a parent? At some point in therapy, I always ask clients to bring in their parents and brothers and sisters. This helps me learn and understand more about them since I can experience them in context. The parents often feel afraid to come into the counseling session, worried that I'm going to jump all over them, blame them for their child's problems, and show them how they were bad parents. Alas and hurrah, things are not that simple. One family of a twenty-four-year-old depressed boy were willing to do everything and anything to help their son. They were terminally understanding, accepting, and helpful, and still he was depressed. As a matter of fact, their totally loving behavior contributed to his staying depressed. What came out in the sessions was that he needed, he *craved*, limits, demands, expectations, appropriate punishment, direction. Their total, loving acceptance left him without the kind of firm experience of support he needed to take on challenges, survive failures, grow, learn, and become autonomous.

There are things you do and say to your kid that you feel simply express love or honesty. Look again. You may find you are subtly undermining your child's self-esteem or independence. One family brought in their twenty-two-year-old son for therapy because he was always depressed, unmotivated, and generally unhappy. He still lived at home, didn't work, and showed enthusiasm or pain only in regard to his girlfriend. The parents' attempts to help their son seemed supportive, but accumulated in the form of subtle undermining. For instance, when after some therapy the son got a job, his father expressed his happiness by saying, "I'm really happy he got this job. It's not a very good one really, and the pay is lousy, but the owner of the business is a schlump who used to work for me and it's a good beginning." Now that touch of honest assessment is real supportive, isn't it? The mother started pressing him for all he should start doing now that he was on the right track and telling him what he should do and feel. That really boosted his self-confidence! This is how you drive your kids crazy.

Has it been brought to your attention by those near and dear to you that you sound just like your overbearing, demanding father or just like your whiny, guilt-provoking mother? How could it happen? You hated it so much when your parents did that to you. You swore you would never behave like them. It's really no mystery. How your parents behaved is your earliest and most powerful role model for how you should act. It's your first schooling in human behavior and you learned it well. Second, and perhaps more important, is that their most miserable behaviors were ones which exerted power over you, made you feel insecure, worthless, powerless. That's why you hated their behaviors. And now you make yourself powerful by gaining the ultimate in acceptance by your parents, and using the tools that had power over you, you become just like your parents. Recognize this pattern and look for ways to become strong and okay in your own style.

Are you disciplining your kids or demoralizing them? A psychologist responding to a TV talk show host's queries on disciplining children said that when your child refuses to eat what you have prepared, you should starve him till the next meal. When he's hungry enough, he'll eat. If eating is the only issue between you and your child that you want to solve, then it will probably work. If issues of respect, understanding, and cooperation are also of interest to you, I think that technique stinks. As an adult, it's all too easy for you to want to make your life convenient. Not to have yet another hassle at home after your hard day. To feel like the boss. To be paranoid about your child's potential for manipulation. But discipline should not have one or more of those as its main driving force. Discipline is not control; it is guidance. If your child truly doesn't like something, find a substitute that you both accept. Find a compromise. One piece of macaroni for five peas. Show a willingness to work it out or you might never see such willingness back.

Did you ever try to pick up warm Jell-O with your fingers? Sometimes being a parent is about as frustrating as that. Your child wants to go to the movies with friends. Maybe in the past you've said "no" immediately and with no explanation. The "no" was to avoid having to think about your fears. Step one to good parenting: Think about those fears, maybe even express them to your children. Tell your child you are worried about transportation and safety, drugs, sex, and whatever else. Step two to good parenting: Give your child the opportunity to respond to your concerns and to find a way to satisfy your rules. In this way, your child might earn your permission. You will discover that some of your fears and concerns are unnecessary, or even excessive. Be willing to accept that. You will discover, too, that in some ways, you have underestimated your child. You will also learn what you do need to teach them or help them with. At this point, you are working together with your child.

Why don't you men spend more time with your kids? All right guys, let's hear the excuses. You work all day and you don't have time. That's what your wife is supposed to do. The kids have their own friends anyway. The bottom line is that both your kids and you are missing out on fun, touching moments, feelings of belonging and loving. You men probably feel competent and comfortable at work, at golf, and in your garage. You might worry about what to say to a little girl, how to hold her without hurting her, how to handle a tantrum or tears. You know, you may be avoiding your kids because you are afraid of looking foolish and clumsy. Parenting is learned. Your wife appears to know more about it because everyone expects her to, so she uses the old trial-and-error way. You male types don't like to look like you don't know what you're doing. So find out. Call your nearest family therapy clinic and join or start a men's parenting workshop and bring the kids.

Are you so sure it's your child who is unreasonable? Making your kids be neat always seems to be important to parents. Well, you want to teach them good habits and you don't want to be inconvenienced by their mess. Maybe, too, you want to feel a sense of power, of respect, by being able to control them. In the latter case, you're going to be at war with your kids, and no one wins that. One mother I was counseling was making her daughter do chores as a way of maintaining the control and importance she silently felt she was losing now that her child was entering adolescence. Once she understood the depth of her own feelings, she could separate out the disciplining from the control. She told her daughter that her room could be whatever she chose it to be but that those areas of the home they shared, they both had to work on keeping neat. The daughter readily agreed. No problem. Make sure you're disciplining, not squeezing.

When you're on your way home from work, what's on your mind? This is where a lot of domestic problems begin, when one of you is on your way home. You're tired and maybe even fed up, especially after hassling with traffic. Your fantasy is to walk through the door and (*a*) not be bothered any further, and (*b*) be repaired by the people in your family already at home. But (*a*) and (*b*) don't come true. You're angry, so you yell, scream, drink, and leave. Let's try something new.

Let's plan a way to make going home an attractant rather than a punishment. Your beloved already at home probably has the same *(a)* and *(b)* fantasies. At some neutral time, talk about those needs, those fantasies, and work out an arrangement that puts you both in the gain column. Some couples meet in the shower, others only after each has had a half hour of time alone. Don't give me or each other excuses about the kids, the terrible day, the dog, or the weather. Make something work so that your marriage will.

Your kid being a rotten little pain? Getting in trouble at school? Stealing from you? Being an almost constant problem? It could be that your child is trying to save you. As a family therapist, I see a lot of parents who bring in their rotten, miserable little kids for me to repair. Often the family wants to leave the child with me and come back when it's all over. I always try to work with the whole family. No, not to find out how the parents messed up their kid. Usually to find out if the child is messing up to help the family in some way. For example, kids find out quickly that being in trouble gets them attention, maybe the kind of attention that distracts the parents from fighting with each other. Kids also discover that being naughty may be the only way to ensure that Mom or Dad takes the opportunity to be an attentive parent. Or to give Mom and Dad the opportunity to relate to each other as though they had something in common. Want to understand your naughty child? Look at the bottom line of what happens from their naughtiness.

Want your child to mind? Give him more than he wants. Many parents come to me frazzled over trying to get their youngster to listen to them. It seems that any child can overpower two competent, strong adults simply by saying "no." Here's how to fight back. When they want something, give them more than they bargained for. Your child wants to stay up later than the bedtime you think is healthy and reasonable? Sure. And you stay up with them, having fun, making sure that little tyke is still awake until the wee hours, till he's begging to go to sleep. Your child wants to have cookies before dinner? Sure, have ten and eat them all. Your child wants to scream, kick, and carry on? Sure. Tape-record it to make sure your child can listen to it, to make improvements, support more tone, volume, range, duration. In other words, with joyful enthusiasm, give 'em what they want and more. They'll back off themselves. And you're not angry and no longer the enemy.

Do you get hurt by your kid's choices and decisions because you take them as reflections on you? One mother came to counseling all upset about her daughter's decision not to have children. At first, she carried on about a woman's role to mother, the responsibility to society, the selfishness of a childless lifestyle, the loneliness of old age without children. These are all worthy arguments. And that's what they were: arguments. The real pain came from her secret fear that her daughter's decision not to have children might mean that her daughter hated her own mothering. This woman felt like a failure. She felt that if her daughter had liked her own family upbringing, she would, of course, want to re-create it in her own life. That is often a factor in decisions, but only one of many factors. Mom hadn't failed as a mother. In fact, her daughter's ability to make up her own mind was a testament to the quality of parenting she got. Your child's very different lifestyle may be a testament to the security you gave them to risk being different.

Do your parents have the power to press your buttons of anger and frustration? Parents always seem to have opinions, criticisms, advice, and suggestions. If you respond to any or all of those with predictable righteous fury, then you're still trapped, and the trap is your demand for unconditional approval. If you think your parents' judgments and expectations are unfair,

how fair is it for you to demand that your folks un-
equivocally approve of your thinking and behaviors?
How fair is it of you to lay on them the guilt trip that
you can't grow up and move on till they agree with
you? Practically speaking, how could you better cope
with their seemingly contrary input? Instead of trying
to convince or convert, why not just appreciate that
they care to be helpful, no matter how they approach
it? Why not thank them, ask questions, savor the information, and then do what you feel is the best for
you and your life? Want your parents to be more tolerant of you? Show 'em how it's done.

Are you competing with and jealous of children? Do
you find yourself resentful of the time, attention, and
affection your beloved shows toward the children?
Before you jump all over your spouse, think about
these questions. Do you find yourself hostile and punitive toward the children with only mild provocation?
Do you find yourself quiet and aloof when the family is
all together? Do you notice how you become rejecting
and critical of your beloved when you two are alone?
If the answers to too many of these were "yes," then a
painful amount of this problem is long-standing within
you. If your early family experiences included quickly
changing allegiances or bartered love, then it's easy to
see how you might be insecure about loving. At this
point in your life it might feel like shared love is lost

love. And that's a tragedy. Don't let this go on. Get some counseling for you and your family. Learn that love naturally expands geometrically.

When you were a child, were you blessed by being given everything you wanted? Are you wondering now if it was more of a curse? It's not unusual for parents to overdo, to want to provide everything for their child, and protect their child from disappointment or hurt, especially if that parent felt deprived as a child. The overdoing came out of love for you and a longing to have had all that themselves. You may have found that you paid a price. The sad outcome of being so overly provided for and overly protected may be that you develop the feeling that all of that had to be done for you because you were unable. The thought becomes reality as you have little experience with trial and error on your own. You may find yourself afraid to make decisions on your own, take risks, try new things. It's not hopeless, but it does take time and guts to move into a place of feeling more confident, to be able to rely on yourself.

Some days are just bummers, and then you go home and what happens? You walk through the front door, and your kids disobey and smart-mouth you. Your beloved isn't being sensitive enough. Your pet is annoyingly bouncy and playful when you want peace. Groan. So you blow up, screaming about what a down coming home has become. Back up a minute. They're probably just being their typical selves and it doesn't always bug you so seriously. So what's happening to you? You need to feel important, useful, and powerful. If you don't get those feelings in one place, you naturally look to another to repair the loss or the damage to your self-esteem. Your family's behavior isn't different or bad; it's just that you're seeing it from an emotionally weather-beaten point of view. What you need, they can't fulfill, so you get angry and impatient. Instead, take a hot bath or run around the block, and then come home and enjoy your family.

I remember one mother who complained about her son's disrespectful loud mouth. "Why, he yells and screams and carries on like a maniac when he doesn't get his own way!" she yelled. After commiserating about how terrible that must be for her, I asked gently where he might have learned that behavior. She screamed at me, "I don't know what's the matter with him! If I knew, I wouldn't be asking you, now would I?" I stayed silent. She got silent—and then said, "Oh."

And with that sigh, she understood immediately that that little rotten creep, her son, was simply mimicking her behavior. So when you want your child's rotten behavior to change, you might have to look into the mirror to begin the process.

Are you taking an exaggerated position in your family relationships? The father of the family rarely involved himself in disciplining the children. When he did, he was a bear, demanding immediate obedience, perfection in all actions, proper respect when speaking to Dad. Whew! The kids were always upset and angry with him. The mom, the more involved parent, was always in the middle. Dad's problem was that he felt guilt for his limited involvement with his children over the years. His work was his life. His feelings of incompetency in parenting came from his lack of experience with his own kids and the jealousy he felt watching his wife be so good at it. His brusque manner, his demandingness, his overrigidity and strictness were his attempts to deny his guilt and feelings of incompetency by literally demanding to be the boss. Your overexaggerated stances are, like this dad's, an attempt to hide your fears, confusions, weaknesses, and mistakes. You have a better chance of rallying your family around you with humility and openness.

Are you worried about your child's developing sense of self-esteem? Parents often want to know what kinds of things they can do to repair or engender a good sense of self in their child. Self-esteem is harder to repair than to originally create, so let's start with the creation. You may think that never saying "no" to your child, never punishing or being angry with them, is the way to help a child build a good self-image. Not so. Children need to learn to adapt to the real world of not always getting their own way, not always being right, and taking responsibility for their actions. My idea of the number-one way to help your child's self-esteem begins and ends with you. The regard a parent shows for himself and his beloved is a powerful experience for a child. One couple never hugged or held each other. Their child was kind of aloof and that worried them. On my suggestion, they snuggled affectionately while their child was playing in the room. As if he were on remote control, he ran over to them and patted their cheeks, laughing with glee. They teared up.

"How do I cope with how tough my husband wants me to be with the kids?" you ask. It's not surprising, considering we all have different family experiences, that parents have different ideas about raising children. I'm always curious, though, about people choosing partners in marriage who they say are the exact opposite of their experience or values. I don't think it's accidental at all. After fifteen years of marriage, this wife was still complaining about her husband's strictness with the kids. Because she was more easygoing and liberal in her disciplining, the kids all showed her more consideration and affection. She came from a family which abused her and valued her brother as the favorite child. With marriage and motherhood, she created a family in which she was now the favorite child because the strict husband had obviously become the bad guy. Is your present discomfort helping you cope with past pain?

How would you react if your husband, the father of your children, told you he was gay? You might feel shocked, angry, hurt, and confused. You might feel used, asking, "Why would you marry me, knowing this about yourself?" Most men are aware of their homosexual feelings from a young age. Many of these men have both homosexual and heterosexual feelings to various degrees, so they're confused, too. These men marry for many reasons: some in the hopes that marriage will eliminate their homosexual feelings, others to comply with family and social expectations, and others to camouflage their homosexuality. Most of you

women might feel that because your husband is homosexual, he couldn't love you, the children or the family, and that's wrong. Your husband, like any other
human being—like you—needs intimacy, commitment,
and family. He could love you emotionally, if not erot-
ically. But what do you both do now? Splitting up is
one option, but not the only one. You both have difficult decisions to make. Take your time and get professional help.

What do you do when you can't please everybody?
Especially around holiday times, you find yourself jug-
gling your schedules around in-laws and relatives,
friends, business associates, and some others you may
not really want to spend time with, but you feel you
should. After all, there are just so many Thanksgiving,
Christmas, and Hanukkah dinners you can eat. You
can't be everywhere with everybody, so what do you
do? It would be easy to say, "Well, I'm just going to do
what I want and the heck with everybody else!" But
the debris from all those hurt feelings would eventually dirty up your pleasure. Instead, be clear on what
your priorities are. Be honest with others about your
situation or predicament. Do something for others in
exchange for their sacrifice in accommodating you.
When you're in a bind, the tendency is to lash out, to
blame or avoid others as though they caused the prob-

lem or could make it go away. You'll have a better holiday if you face this situation with honesty, sensitivity, and compromise.

Don't make the process of changing become a war. One lady I'm counseling began to understand the origins of her reluctance to behave like a mother instead of a buddy or a child to her adolescent daughter. When she finally decided she was worthy and competent to assume the mother role, she did so with a vengeance, hitting her daughter with a backlog of fifteen years of parental rules, restrictions, demands, and commands. Suddenly, mother and daughter were at war. When Mom spoke with me, she complained about her daughter's lack of immediate cooperation and acquiescence to this new reality. She was hurt and angry, seeing in her daughter the enemy, keeping Mom from making things right. If things have been a certain way, it's been with everyone's cooperation and acceptance. For better or worse, the ground rules were set. Everyone obeyed. You were allies. To make a change work well, you must all be allies in the transition, respecting each other's confusion, loss, and pain. Without that, growth becomes torture instead of revelation.

Having in-law problems? You know you are handling your in-law problems wrong when the problem never seems to get better. If you are having difficulty with an in-law who is too intrusive, who is divisive and destructive to your marriage, consider the following: The pattern was most likely set down long before you entered the picture. That means that you didn't cause it and you probably aren't, therefore, going to be able to fix it. In-law problems are really problems in that original family. You've married into it. Your spouse may allow you to get all upset and fight it out so that he or she doesn't have to. In this way, your spouse is continuing to protect his parents from his *own* pain and hostility. That's loving, but *you* become the hit man. Don't fight it out with the in-law, don't set down laws for your spouse's behavior with his or her own parent. Do require and solicit your spouse's loyalty and primary attachment. Your spouse has to mature to the point of leaving home—his first one.

Why is it that there's no place like home? After a few weeks of the job, the kids, the house, the bills, the noise, the problems, you begin to dream of nothing else but getting away, so you go away. You have fun, unwind. In the midst of all that refreshing R and R, you begin to dream of nothing else but going home. Certainly, you're not dreaming of the problems, yet there's something special about home. You're amused at the behavior of dogs marking trees, fences, and posts with their own scent. You may not be aware of how much of that behavior is important to you. You mark out your territory, too. You have your special things in their special places, some of which have wonderful memories. Others are convenient. All spell comfort, familiarity, and security. Home is your anchor, your launch pad, your recovery room, your playpen, your womb. In a world of relentless challenges, threats, hurts, and insecurity, home offers an umbilicus to a long-lost sense of total safety. Be it ever so frazzled, there's no place like home.

# CHAPTER 2

# *Relationships*

Remember that last argument you had with your dearly beloved? It's possible that you were both right. You may be more used to arguments that are resolved by finding out, proving, making one person seem right and the other wrong. The point is to win the argument as the means of ending it. The arguing may stop on the surface. The hurt feelings may continue to fester under the surface. A better way of ending arguments is to resolve the issues and feelings aroused. This can be done only if you are willing to accept the validity of the other person's feelings. That their feelings might be different from yours does not invalidate your feelings. Your defensiveness in response to their expressions of pain, anger, or disappointment may come from your feelings of guilt or competitiveness for the position of the person wronged. Listen to your partner's version of the situation and try to feel what it would be like to see it their way. There's no better enticement to have them do the same for you.

How do you know for sure that someone cares about you? Well, let's see. You might assume someone cares about you if you generally are treated well. It's nice when you get verbal assurances, too, and you may or may not require that. But what if you get verbal assurances but *aren't* generally treated well? That's tricky. Your partner's saying the right thing and sometimes doing the wrong thing. How do you judge someone's caringness then? Their caringness is not the issue. What you want and need as a person is the issue. If you are feeling jerked around emotionally, that's what's probably happening to you. You stay in such a relationship and struggle for the other to change certain behaviors toward you because of feelings inside *you*. You probably don't feel lovable. So you gratefully accept your partner's protestations of caring amidst their cruelty. You are all too tolerant of it. The person whose caring toward you I am most concerned with is you.

Ever notice that there are times when you seem to almost grit your teeth and refuse to be sexually turned on to your beloved? Feelings of sensuality and sexuality are quite natural to the experience of being human.

Being held, caressed, and stimulated brings about sexual arousal. You can recognize those times when you simply refuse to allow that to happen. What's that about? Sometimes you refuse to allow your partner to be physically loving to you because you're still angry over some unresolved conflict. This is your silent punishment: not giving of yourself. It may be that you're so absorbed in the painful, stressful aspects of your life that you reject your beloved as a way of weakly striking back at the world, or your denying yourself pleasure is part of your sadness and frustration. Whatever the motivation, your loss of the physical warmth is so great a price to pay. Babies, puppies, kittens, and you thrive on physical closeness with the pleasure and reassurance it brings. When things get the worst, the worst is to lose touch.

What's so good about a committed relationship anyway? Lots of you in committed relationships are walking around feeling oppressed, tied down, taken for granted. You daydream about freedom and flexibility. You may even test that out. Yet, be it ever so humble, you always go home. What is it really in your relationship that makes you feel so constricted? Is it that your partner knows you so well, faults and flops? Does that embarrass and anger you? On the other hand, where else are you so safe to be so real? Some new person can do a temporary puffing up of your ego, but you might become wary of showing too much of yourself lest someone's fantasy bubble about you burst. It might be that you feel constricted in your relationship because your own rigidity is in the way. Your notion of rules and roles might be the true culprit. How frank are you about your needs, wishes, and desires? How tolerant are you of your beloved's? Maybe the new exciting territory of romance and joy to explore is at home.

"I'll never let anyone close enough to hurt me again!" If you've gone through considerable emotional pain, risked vulnerability, and felt hurt, abused, or betrayed for your trouble, it's not unreasonable for you to feel cautious. Perhaps being more careful about your choice of people or your pacing of intimacy would be a good idea. If your statement of "never again" is a temporary reaction to your hurt and fear, some amount of backing off might be good for you. You could use this time to think things through. However, if your statement is more of a commitment to isolation, please stop for a moment and consider the consequences. Not letting anyone close to you ever again because you've been hurt is like using steel windows in a house to keep out the dust. It works; steel windows will keep the dust out. Also the smell of spring flowers, birds and children chirping, and cool reassuring breezes.

Not letting people close to you keeps you from being hurt by them; then the only source of your hurt is yourself.

Do you have a compulsive spouse? Is your spouse too industrious, too perfectionist, and too demanding? Do you feel lazy or incompetent by comparison? Do you feel left out and unimportant? Before you were married, you probably saw your hardworking spouse as dependable and secure. Your spouse may have seen your easygoing manner as a welcome relief from an earlier, overdemanding atmosphere. But now your spouse is compulsive, selfish, and insensitive, and you're a lazy unappreciative nag, right? You two didn't marry by accident. Your spouse saw in you someone who was nondemanding, nonthreatening, and controllable. You saw in your spouse someone you could depend on and blame for just about everything. Neither one of you is right or wrong. You both need to evolve. Your spouse needs to trust someone else with his emotional vulnerability so that staying in control won't be such a frenzied necessity, and you need to become more self-respecting and sufficient so that you can share, not lean.

Why is it so easy for people to grow apart? When you are estranged, it's easy to say, "Well, it just happens like that sometimes. People grow apart." That's implying that relationships come and go with the wind, subject to the whim of the fates. Actually, you aren't an innocent bystander. You are a participant. Maybe you grow apart from someone when you can't forgive him for not living up to your fantasy of a lover and a partner. Instead, you find fault and disgust in his true personhood. Maybe you grow apart from someone when he doesn't cater to your whims and moods, always making you feel better. Maybe you grow apart from someone because she needs to grow and change in ways that threaten your ego or security. Maybe you grow apart from someone because she needs you in ways you feel inadequate or frightened to fulfill. Maybe you grow apart from someone because he wants you to be more vulnerable and open, and you're scared to death.

Do you have a tough time letting go? The image that comes to my mind is your hanging on to your telephone receiver long after the other person has hung up. Somehow, if you don't hang up your end, you can feel as if the conversation, perhaps even the relationship, isn't over. There is a sense of finality when the circle is complete. You may be doing irrational things just to keep from accepting the reality that something in your life has ended. When you do accept it, you'll feel an unexpected sense of relief. A relief from holding back your feelings, holding up denial, and holding forth useless hope. When you're swamped with emotional pain and a crumbled self-esteem, moving on may seem too frightening. Holding on protects you from the imagined hobgoblins of your mind. Think of monkey bars, like when you were a kid, dangling up there, straining to get the next bar with one hand, holding on for dear life with the other. When both hands held their targets, you had a moment's choice to go back or forward. Make that decision now.

Are you banging on a wall, trying to turn it into a door? Think about it. How many times have you tried telling, yelling, asking, begging, demanding that people to do or be someone they can't or won't do or be? How many times have you sacrificed everything for the sake of something with little or no percentage of return? Some may call you perseverant, but I don't. I call you frightened. When you want someone who's kind, attentive, and affectionate and you feel lovable and competent in relationships, you go out and find someone just like that. You don't try to change a cold, withdrawn, argumentative person into one. No, you do that when the end product, the kindness and affection, scares you in some way. Being stuck with what you don't want is the way you keep yourself safe from

what it is you do want, but which scares or threatens
you. If you're stuck with a dud, or you are in a pickle,
don't complain about your fate, the dud, or the pickle.
Find out what it is about your dream that you fear.

Are you married to an emotional hit man? I worked
with a perfect family once, at least that's what the
mother kept saying. "My husband is wonderful. My
daughter is wonderful. My son is wonderful. It's just
that he married a miserable witch who keeps him
from calling and seeing me." That her son would
break the tradition of "wonderfulness" and marry a
virtual hit man, someone who shows anger and tells
the family off, is not an accident. Families have rules
and rituals, some of which *are* wonderful, like dinners
together and open family conferences. However, some
of the rules are stifling and destructive, even when the
original intentions were benevolent. Expectations
such as "We look good at all costs" or "Negative words
or feelings are never allowed" obstruct individuality
and true family mutuality. This son married a hit lady
as a compromise between the enforced "wonderfulness" of his family and his need to show his true feelings. If your children's behaviors go against the family
grain, look more closely at the grain before you complain.

Do you hesitate to tell your dearly beloved about a problem for fear of worrying them? One man said he'd been out of work a month and just got a new job, but hadn't told his wife about this whole trial and tribulation. "I just didn't want to upset or worry her," he said, so magnanimously. There are times when telling our intimates our troubles is more burdening them than informing or recruiting them in some useful way, but it's not always the case. I asked him if he thought he knew his wife well. He said, "Yes." I asked him if he thought she would have been pleased or relieved not to be involved in his pain or fearful difficulties. His voice dropped into his shoes as he said, "Well, no." I asked him if he feared or distrusted her. He said, "No." And I wondered why he would hide from her at a time when he needed her and she could have responded to his need. "I was afraid she would think I was a failure. I was afraid she would stop loving me." Since he thought he was a failure, he thought she would think that, so he avoided her. This kind of avoidance creates a void between people. Share it and survive together.

Who is your worst enemy? One lady thought her husband was her worst enemy. "He never does me favors anymore. He's always angry and snippy and we fight all the time." This young woman and her husband were both twenty-five years old, married six years with a one-year-old child. Was it an interesting coincidence that the tensions appeared about a year and a half ago? No. These people moved from their childhood homes into a marital situation, their freedom further diminished by their responsibility for a child. Destiny seemed to be set in cement shoes. Both felt afraid, trapped, and frustrated. Both felt guilt for these feelings. Both couldn't face the feelings or the guilt. Both found something more tangible and safe to be angry about—each other. When you're working up to being angry with each other, you find things to justify your anger, anything from tone or facial expressions to small mistakes. The fights are brusque, but superficial. Nothing's resolved. Feelings are hurt. Relationships and people destroyed. Get some help to face the real problems.

Where do you draw the line between your needs and your partner's needs? There are two important elements to this question. First, to distinguish between true needs and indiscriminate, manipulative demands. Second, not to look at give-and-take moment by moment, but as a trend over time. Sometimes what you or your partner expresses as a need is more of a demand whose intent is to challenge, test, or control, in which case you might choose to be responsive because of guilt, fear, or a lack of a sense of limit on what ought to be expected of a person. Other times, you or your partner might indeed make unreasonable, even hysterical demands, which might be met out of compassion or momentary expediency. If most of your reaction to your partner's needs is out of a sense of expediency, you've sold yourself down the river. Relationships that are not reciprocal are resentful. The price for not feeling a sense of being caretaken as you caretake is a feeling of loneliness and anger.

How can you ensure that as the years go by, you grow together with your loved one and not apart? Since you can only be responsible for and orchestrate your end of the relationship, since you could change, since life is unpredictable, you can't plan the future in minute detail. You must be able to accept these realities without constant hiccups of insecurity, which are deadly to relationships. You've got to think of togetherness as your involvement in your beloved's life, and not only their attention to yours. You've got to temper your raging expectations of total immersion in each other as the only acceptable state if the relationship is going to work at all. I know it's romantic to say, "Ah, my love, we are now one." But the separateness is a physical truth and is to be respected as an often emotional necessity. You've got to expect and accept the reality of change. That person you picked to commit your life and soul to is going to evolve. Not only do you need to let them, you must support them in it.

Do you have a spouse who never seems to stop working? You nag, beg, complain, threaten, all to no avail. They never seem to have time for fun, time for the two of you. Such compulsiveness is often an indication of unconscious fears. Your spouse may feel deep inside that without working, he will not get the rewards of love and approval. Arguing about something largely unconscious is not very useful. You already know that, so sneak in. Instead of complaining about how much your spouse does, start rewarding him for his efforts. If he complains that he shouldn't be rewarded because the task isn't totally completed or because there is so much else to do, tell him, "I know you're not done, but you certainly deserve a reward for how much you've done so far." Compliments, plaques, back rubs, special goodies—try whatever works and keep it up. The hope is that your spouse will finally and unconsciously accept your efforts as more reasonable than the cruel parenting he's been imposing on himself.

Are you where you are out of want or need? I was watching a deeply moving film the other day in which a mother, dying of cancer, was trying to give her daughter freedom from guilt and a secret stash of money so the girl could leave the small town and start her own adult life. Her mother explained that she had accumulated the money early in the marriage to the girl's father so that she always had the means to leave. On the girl's way to the bus station, she says good-bye to her dad, who also tries to give her whatever money he has on him. She refuses, saying she already has enough. Her dad replies, "Oh, Mom gave you her private stash, huh?" When the girl looks surprised at his knowledge of the money, he responds gently, "Oh, I've always known about it, and I've always felt proud and filled with joy because I knew your mom stayed with me because she wanted me, and not because she couldn't go." I'm not convinced you can truly love if you can't separate out what you deeply want from what you fearfully cling to.

Are you and your beloved behaving like emotional orthodontists? I remember going to the orthodontist to get braces on my bottom teeth. First, he had to pull out a perfectly good, but crammed-in tooth. Then he had to put those little rubber spacers in between my teeth to spread them out. After the spacers did their torturous job, my teeth were wide apart enough to put the braces on. You and your dearly beloved may be performing orthodontics on your relationship all the time and finding that the relationship is not straightening out at all. Picking, nagging, oversensitivity, fights over "gosh, I don't remember" are all spacers to separate you and your beloved from each other. "But why would I do that?" you ask so innocently. Think about it. If you hadn't had that fight, what might have happened instead? Maybe this will help you discover what you're avoiding. Might you have had sex? Maybe you would have been vulnerable, asking for help or admitting to some fears. You might have been found out to be naughty or incorrect. What do those fights help you to avoid?

Are you sure you're not being cared about? "I expect you to do for me as I am willing to do for you" is not a fair or productive comment. You may be feeling unloved, uncared for, because your loved ones and friends are not giving and doing for you exactly what you are giving and doing for them. Remember now, love can be expressed in different languages. My friend's notion of making a statement about our closeness is to jump up whenever I want something and go get it for me. My notion of showing the same sentiment is to let her help herself to whatever she would like in my home. If we didn't clarify our feelings and intent, we'd both probably feel hurt all the time. The important part in adjusting to someone close is not to have her or you adopt the other person's language, although one or both of you might enjoy doing that in some areas. The important part is to be open with each other about your feelings, your interpretations, and your intent. Without that step of openness, you will both be treading water in a turbulent lake of misunderstanding.

"Hey, it's not my problem. It's your problem." "I'm going to do what I'm going to do. You don't like it, that's your problem." Whoa, do you hear that a lot? Worse yet, do you say that a lot? When two people are close, caring, and mutually involved, how can there be a one-sided or one-dimensional problem? If loved ones are going to have some trouble coping or accepting your words or deeds, what good does it do you to leave them emotionally stranded to work it out or eat it alone? Their unhappiness or their rebellion will impinge upon you sooner or later. I think you may flaunt that "your problem" attitude when you're not so sure of yourself. Because if you dump everything on them, you don't have to examine much about yourself that could stand some examining. If you've been angry or hurt and feeling vengeful, this might be an ideal way for you to exert power and control and tell 'em to "Stick it!" Stay in each other's lives, share the problem.

Does your dearly beloved seem unreasonably jealous? If so, it's time to do something about it. Think about how you do contribute to your beloved's feelings of insecurity. For instance, you may be more involved in work, friends, or sports than ever before, you may be sharing your intimate thoughts less and less, you may have withdrawn sexually—and you may not be aware of any of this. Your partner may be picking up on what might be your subtle acts of distancing and rejection. So before your partner gets labeled an annoying, jealous creep, consider that you might be causing your beloved to feel less loved, valued, and wanted by you. Figure out what's bothering you—finances, sex, children, health, work, boredom—whatever. Realize that some of your behaviors which are driving your partner into "jealous" reaction are your way of avoiding things going on in you and between you. Honesty, reassurance, and compassion go a long way in curing this kind of jealousy.

There are times when you use honesty as an excuse for controlling and hurting your partner. Here's an example: One woman wondered about her husband's immature jealousy because, she said, "He gets all upset when I tell him about being excited by other men. I tell him only to be honest about my thoughts and feelings. And my thoughts and feelings are perfectly natural." Now, that's just not true. She was telling him of her roving eye and raging hormones to test him, control him, hurt him, and make him feel insecure. The next time you are debating whether or not to tell your partner the truth, think first of your intent. Do you have any possible hidden, ulterior motives? You might be hurting that someone you're supposed to care about to keep from revealing your fears or needs. Instead, you use being able to cause pain or emotional discomfort as a most unpleasant way of reassuring yourself of your power.

You meet somebody new. It's so exciting, so spontaneous. It seems you don't even have to work at it—for a while. Be honest. Do you really think support, physical and emotional intimacy, safety and comfort can come free? What you do get from a love relationship is an opportunity to create all those possibilities for yourself. Finding someone to do that with is a gift of a lifetime. What work is required? It's giving. No, I don't mean gifts and other assorted goodies. It is the giving of your time, attention, vulnerabilities, needs, thoughts, feelings, dreams, fears, and hopes, and that's the work you might fear and avoid doing. The so-called hard work that a relationship really needs is nothing more and nothing less than the depth of you yourself. That means—and here's the punch line—the work you have to do in a relationship is the same work you have to do for your own personal growth.

Does your partner tell you that you are just too hard to please and nothing is ever good enough for you? And do you snarl back, "That's a cop-out, dear"? Look again. Try to figure out how you could have picked out someone like that, someone so far from your expectations of how a partner should be. And if you've made a mistake, why browbeat them over it? Also, look at how reasonable your demands and expectations really are. It's obvious that you are tormenting others with your expectations of them. Maybe it's not so obvious to you that you are tormenting yourself even more. If your rigid, perfectionistic, demanding expectations are never met, you never have anything to enjoy. You lose out. Each of your many unmet expectations is another addition to your unhappiness. Frankly, I would hate to be unable to enjoy a good Italian dinner just because it's short a few spaghetti strands.

Have you ever said, "If he does that one more time, I'll go nuts"? Here's a suggestion about how to save your sanity: Realize three things. One, the behavior, as infuriating as it is to you, means something very important to your partner. For example, neatness may be his attempt to feel in control of something in his life. Two, the behavior, since it is a habit, just happens automatically. Do not think it is a premeditated plan to irk you. Three, the behaviors are rooted in early childhood experiences and are very difficult to stop or change. So what can you do? Try to see it from his vantage point. Telling him to stop straightening things up is not as effective as helping him face and understand the discomforts or anxieties that drive him to those repetitive, annoying behaviors. Fighting him doesn't help you, helping him will.

Should you ever give him a last chance, and then one more time? Yes, sometimes you should give one more chance past the last one—when there is enough information to suggest to you that you can only gain. Forgiving ad nauseam has no power to seduce or induce people to change. It just gives you the opportunity to xerox the disappointment and pain. If you're going to give yet another chance, a few things ought to be made clear. One, that there are certain specific conditions—call them acts of good faith—that must be met. These conditions need to be efforts which require real physical, psychological, or moral exertion. And two, that their getting another chance does not mean that you are compromising on those conditions. Why should you give another chance at all? Because it might be better for you in the long run to get what you really want—what would make you better off—rather than get short-term revenge but not end up with your goodies.

How come love doesn't always feel loving? The end of the fairy tale always promises, "And they lived happily ever after." It was like that in the beginning for you, too. But now you sometimes awaken in the night, look over at your partner, and wonder who that is. Your heart pounds as you watch your television hero or heroine. You look over at your partner and you don't feel that same rush. All in all, you are sure you two have lost love. Chances are, what you've lost is your perspective on love. Books and movies often present love only in the framework of passion, excitement, and mystery. These are lovers' games. You can always play, and I suggest you do. But don't forget the elements of love that can't be had on a first meeting, no matter how thrilling. You won't have acceptance for yourself, the sharing of dreams finally coming true. The understanding that comes only through time. The history of successes enjoyed and failures survived. Real life.

If your partner is asking you to give up your life's ambitions, your ethics, morality, your deep desire to have children, your relationship with your family, your education, or anything else of serious moment, then you need to consider carefully his motivations and your welfare. But if your partner is asking you to give up late working hours, drinking, a sedentary lifestyle, a secretive aloof demeanor, or other such compulsive but not constructive aspects of your lifestyle, then you need to consider carefully your motivations for refusing. Let's hear the excuses. "How dare you tell me what to do? You're trying to control me! You're stealing my identity." Some of the changes you're being asked to make may be good ones for you and necessary for the relationship. Protecting rotten habits just because they're yours is a commitment to rejection and loneliness.

There's a famous quote from a movie called *Love Story:* "Love is never having to say you're sorry." I think that's a dangerous philosophy. There are times, even with your loved ones and close friends, when in anger you say the wrong thing. That generally means you have misused something you know that other person is vulnerable to, something she's shared with you in the safe context of your intimate friendship. It might be one of those things that make a permanent scar, not so much because of what you said, but because you dared to fight so dirty with someone you cared about, who trusted you. It's the breach of trust that hurts the most. If you now rely on taking it for granted that they'll understand about the heat of the battle and forgive you automatically, forget it. You are helping erect a silent wall between the two of you. Your only hope is to say that you're sorry, over and over again, acknowledging the breach and the damage. Love means always saying you're sorry.

Lots of you women are complaining that your men are not sensitive enough to your feelings. Lots of you men are wondering what you can do to be more sensitive to your women's feelings. First, to you women. When you complain to your men, do you do it as a critical attack (guaranteed to get further withdrawal)? Are you specific enough? Do you say, "I'd like you to hold my hand when we walk"? Or do you vaguely hit him with, "How come you never pay any attention to me?" A lot of getting what you want hinges on your knowing what you want and being willing to ask for it kindly and directly. And now to you men. The true key to being more sensitive to a woman's feelings is to be honest with yourself and her that you have tender and sensitive feelings. Sensitivity touches sensitivity. If you don't allow yourself to touch and share those parts of yourself, how do you expect to recognize or deal with them in your woman?

What's your bottom line? The term "commitment" is used in so many different ways. Some of you see it as the ultimate in a trap or the loss of privacy and self-determination. Others of you see it as the ultimate in security and safety. Many of you try to define it in such a way as to maximize your own personal flexibility. In your own intimate relationship, you may be behaving as though commitment were a continually negotiable commodity depending upon your mood, your opportunities, your need to threaten; the loss of it as a weapon of anger. The relationships which last see in a commitment the bottom line "I'd rather be with this person than not." Once that is established in your mind, it helps guide you in making decisions which could jeopardize your bottom line. If you're going to be filled with resentment every time you feel you had to give up something so important because of your commitment, remind yourself of your bottom line.

Feel used and abused in your relationship? Many of you give, give, and give some more only to end up feeling spent and lonely. You suffer, then pick yourself up and try all over again. Down deep inside, you are just certain that continual giving is eventually going to get you the love and respect you yearn for. The frustration is that it doesn't ever seem to work out that way. But you are perseverant, so you just keep trying as though it somehow were your responsibility. You need to do more, better, longer. Your abundant giving is being accepted by those who have abundant need. Those are the people least likely to be able to give back, and that is the problem you can't solve by giving more, better, or longer. Keep in mind that you don't have to finish giving before you can receive. It's all right to receive for your very willingness to give, for whatever you have already given. This means you need to focus your giving on those whose need to receive is as great as their need to give.

I've got a surefire method for you to win every argument with your dearly beloved. You see, up to now, you've probably tried to win arguments by going on the opposite side of her position. Annoyingly, she tends to stay on her side as you try to yank her onto your side. If you score what you think is a win, you get punished for it later, nullifying it. You'll agree, this is no fun at all. Well, I have a surefire technique for winning each and very argument: beat her at her own game. If you want to go to the movie once a week, but your partner complains that you both only do what *you* want, fool 'em! Make an agreement to even it up; then you'll get your once-a-week movie. Aha! If your partner says you're only affectionate when you want sex, so your partner usually says "no" to sex, fool 'em! Be affectionate almost all of the time in all sorts of little ways. Then sex will sort of happen as a mutual surprise. Trust me, this works. The less you give your partner to fight about, the more you win.

Maybe you're mad at the wrong person! Are you angry with the neighbor who serves too many drinks to your husband, or an in-law who's always rude to you even though your spouse says you're too sensitive, or an acquaintance who always asks your beloved to do things just at the time you want him to do something together? Sound familiar? Notice a pattern? Your beloved never seems to have any responsibility for actions. It's as though everyone else has the power to be a puppeteer, determining your beloved's behaviors. It's just that you never seem to get your hands near the strings. There really isn't much to lose being angry with outsiders, but there might be too much to lose with a beloved—attachment, affection, attention. So with the fear of that much to lose, you fight dragons for your life, and yet you still feel your life is dripping away. It doesn't have to be all-out war, but it is a risk. Yet to make any progress toward more intimacy and security, you've got to go direct to the source: your beloved.

Not sure if you should get married? So many times I get letters describing the intended spouse and asking, "Should I marry him or her?" As a therapist, it isn't my place to make decisions for you, but I can offer some ideas for you to add to your own decision making. Picking a partner is a complex phenomenon. It involves dreams and fantasies, unresolved emotional issues, practical considerations, pressures, fears, needs. When some of these are not fulfilled, the disappointment too often turns into depression and rage. If you are debating about marriage, perhaps this will help. Consider whether marriage is an addition to what you are building in your life from yourself, or whether marriage is a substitute for your own personal development. In the additive mode, you have much to offer. In the substitutive mode, you have much potential disappointment and frightened dependency. Which marriage do you think has the better chance?

Do you just hate your jailer of a spouse? Many of you probably could complain forever about your controlling, demanding, critical spouse. It's likely that friends and relatives are most compassionate. They take your side and even tell you to dump that mean and rotten person. Yet you don't. You suffer on, explaining that you don't leave because of love. Maybe you stay because deep down inside you know that your spouse is your biggest protector. By being negative, critical, and controlling, your spouse gives you permission to allow your fears to go unnoticed as the real reason you don't go out and work or train or socialize. If you felt secure or worthy enough to be involved in life in a more outgoing way, you wouldn't have picked that particular person to be your spouse. Nor would you have fought trying, really trying, to change the situation. If you really want things to be different in your life, start with thanking your spouse for taking the heat off your fears.

What should you do about the other woman's attempts to continue communicating with your husband after their affair is over? Without deep, basic trust, there is no intimacy. Trust is definitely compromised when you painfully discover your husband has had an affair, no matter how brief. Trusting again requires two main parts: your frank decision to do just that—trust—and your husband's obvious efforts to demonstrate to you that your decision to trust is respected. That means if the other woman continues to contact your husband, you must leave it up to him to handle that problem with resolute firmness. If he is not following through, then it might mean he has mixed feelings or he really hasn't ended it. At least you know you've given this painful predicament the best chance you could. If you're not satisfied that the effort is being returned, then the other woman's existence is secondary to the fragile existence of your relationship.

You think that you and your partner are almost bitter enemies. It's likely that you are secretly protecting each other. So many times people come into therapy certain that one or the other is at fault, is mean, or whatever. Here's an example of what unravels. One man came into therapy alone, saying that his wife was sexually cold. When I met with the couple, a fascinating interaction became obvious. He had experienced some problems with impotency at a stressful time in his life. She had tried to be kind and helpful by not pushing him to perform sexually because she didn't want to see him as upset as he got when he could not function. He read this as rejection, which made the impotency problem worse. His view was that she was cold and rejecting. The underlying dynamic was that she was trying to protect him from failure. Look again at your predicament with someone close. Can you imagine a way in which those behaviors you dislike so much could possibly be an attempt at loving?

Do you sometimes say, "I feel," followed by "that you're being mean to me"? Or "that you don't love me"? That's cheating. When you preface descriptions or complaints about people with "I feel," you are robbing them of their right to disagree. How can anyone argue about your feelings? Well, they can't. It's sacred ground. Irrefutable. Be fair. If you are asking a question, ask it. If you are making a complaint, make it. If you want to talk about your feelings, keep it all about yourself. Here's an example. Let's say you're wanting more attention. "I'm feeling needy of some hugging from you." Now that's honest, vulnerable, and a good use of your feelings.

Are you having an affair? At this moment, you're feeling either caught and guilty or innocent and holy. If you're not involved sexually with another than your spouse, you're not off the hook yet. Extrarelational sex is not the only affair possible. Consider that the end result of an affair is that your attention and affection go elsewhere. Many of you wives are having affairs with your kids, although you rationalize your overinvolvement with the children to the exclusion of your husband as motherhood. And many of you men are having affairs with work, puttering, or viewing sports. You rationalize your overinvolvement as responsibility, R and R, or manly rights. When it comes right down to it, the corespondent in your affair is not as important as the fact that you're running away from problems in the relationship, solving only your end of the problem by distracting yourself. Now answer the question: Are you having an affair? If so, realize that the pain it causes your beloved is the same as if it were sexual. It's the loss of you.

How do you know when your relationship is over? It would be a lot easier to know when your relationship is finished and done if there were some obvious signs, like no more feelings at all or the other person becoming all bad in your eyes. Well, you know you can try to ignore your feelings, or you can try to paint your ex-to-be as all bad, but it's not the truth. There are no tangible end points. There is only your decision: your decision to terminate the relationship and cope with lingering feelings of longing or fond nostalgic moments of the way it was when it was good. Don't mistake those feelings or memories for some omen that you should stay in the relationship. They are simply part of the reality of human experience. Relationships end when you decide to stop trying to be interested, compassionate, tolerant, vulnerable, and involved. Remember, the relationship may end, but those feelings, memories, and longings for love don't end as quickly. Give yourself time.

Maybe the problem in your relationship is that you don't trust your partner. You may not realize that trusting is your problem. Not telling your partner of certain thoughts, feelings, needs, and wants is a way of not trusting. You may alibi by saying, "She's too nervous to deal with this stuff," or, "He's got too many things on his mind." The truth is that you're afraid of how you might be judged and punished. That's the child's mind in you thinking of your partner as your parent. The adult's mind in you has to take risks of self-disclosure and exposure. Working through feelings on that level makes for the kind of intimacy that allows for better sex, communication, and comfortable companionship. After all, if you can't trust your partner with the truth, how can you trust her with the rest of you? Oh, I know what you're thinking. If I start telling what I think, feel, and want, there'll be such a storm. Maybe you're right. Remember, after storms comes a rainbow.

How do you decide what kind of gift to buy someone? You've probably had the opportunity to say, or maybe hear, those fateful words: "Oh, thank you. How lovely. Just what I've always wanted. Mumble, mumble, mumble." Why is it that you make mistakes in giving gifts? You've spent the time and the money, but you were off target. Or were you? I'm convinced that you were on target. It's just that the target was not matching the gift to the person. The target you hit right on was the one with hidden meaning. You may have given that gift as a hint of what you'd like the person to be, like when you gave a flamboyant nightie to your rather conservative lady. You may have given that gift because it's what you'd like. Maybe you hoped that the gift would impress, intimidate, or even punish. There are lots of maybes here, but it's no maybe that you are not considering the true desires and tastes of that person.

Be careful being too helpful to friends in need. Need is one of the greatest seductions. When someone is all pouty-lipped and teary-eyed, with hands outstretched, palms upward, it's so difficult to do other than offer a helping hand. Because he's apparently hurting so much and it feels so good to be in the position of being strong, supportive, and helpful, you go all out to do whatever, whenever, at any cost of time, effort, and privacy. Then you find yourself feeling as though you're filling a bottomless pit of need. The resentment begins. Then the confusion. Then the anger. You end up rejecting that person and adding a feeling of betrayal to his already hurting psyche. Helping does not mean to provide all that the other appears to be needing. That makes you a necessary, permanent fixture if that person is to stay happy. Helping means to provide understanding and support as he goes about devising new ways to get his needs met.

"This relationship is hopeless! But I just can't let go of what little we have." Do you find yourself separated, but never divorced? Or forever living at the edge of breaking up, or never quite letting go after the divorce? You may not realize that the two of you have found a safe medium between what appears to be frightening about too much intimacy and what appears to be frightening about too much aloneness.

Perhaps when you're together, you're driven to obtain or create something impossible in your togetherness. That frantic imperative is permitted rest only when there is the space of threatened dissolution between you. You no longer expect or demand because you're not really together. This may be more appealing than when you both hassle each other to pieces. If it is the alternative of choice, so be it. If it is the alternative of fear, confusion, or helplessness, don't let it be. Give yourself the opportunity to learn how to allow yourself more and get some help with it.

Give someone a gift today. Are you spending too much time worrying about keeping the score even? "He didn't do this or that for me, so I'm not going to give him this or do that for him." Terrific attitude. Certain to breed goodwill. Guaranteed to cheer up your day. There is an interesting *Star Trek* episode in which Captain Kirk finally figured out that this evil, alien creature was living off bad feelings, like hate, resentment, mistrust, and vengeance. So he had everyone spreading cheer no matter how they felt or what had come before. Of course, the evil alien creature evaporated and all was well. Real life not so simple, you say? Be more selective as to the where and with whom and be more intent with the how, I say. Try giving some small but well-meaning—even undeserved— gifts. I don't mean something purchased. I mean something offered with personal sensitivity: a hug, compliments, something repaired, something made, a task taken care of. There's fun in it. It's an icebreaker. It may be the beginning.

# CHAPTER 3

# *Communicating*

Have you ever said, "You can take that any way you'd like; you will anyway"? You've probably said that in a burst of intolerable frustration, thinking that the other is twisting your words into unintentional meanings just to stick it to you. Now, take a deep breath and relax. Two things I want to check out with you. One, that some percentage of your unconscious, unspoken meaning might have been picked up correctly. Ouch! And, two, that you are not being sensitive to what your words might mean to someone else. Not everyone grows up with the same emotional meanings attached to the same words. To some, being called "cute little munchkin" is a sign of affection. To others, the same name might feel like a putdown. Saying you communicate because you say what's on your mind is not enough for an award. You've got to clarify that what you say conveys the same meaning to other people. They aren't twisting your meanings. They're clarifying what your words mean to them. You need to respect that with compassion.

Are you sure your communication problem isn't really a convincing problem? You parents worry about having communication problems with your children. Is it that they or you can't or won't be open? Or is it that you both want the other to acquiesce or agree to the other's point of view? You spouses complain about communication problems with each other, too. You figure that since your words didn't change the other's mood or sentiments, you two don't communicate. Let's straighten this out now. Good communication means that each of you is willing to be frank and clear and will listen and acknowledge the words and feelings of the other. That definition says nothing about convincing the other to change. The biggest communication problems arise when you are not willing to share or you are not willing to accept the other's point of view or feelings. Your openness makes you vulnerable. Your acceptance makes you tolerant. Both make you a good communicator and a very lovable person.

Do you listen or just hear the echo? Listening is a tricky business. People use words. You could just listen to that. People use tones and inflections. You could interpret their words through that. And then

there is the echo, the visceral feeling of their words re-
sounding through the caverns of your memories,
fears, and feelings. That's the hardest listening to do.
One woman couldn't hear her husband, only his echo.
When he told her his feelings about her weight problem, he said, "Darling, I love you and respect you, and
sometimes your weight bothers me a lot and sometimes not. I'd prefer you to lose it, but it doesn't
change my love for you." She, however, heard him say
that he'd never loved her and their life together was a
humiliating lie. She heard it that way because his
words echoed through the halls of her low self-esteem
and fears of not being loved. That's an easy trap to fall
into. It's hard to listen to the truth of someone close to
you when you have your own, frightful feelings and
fears. Remember, though, getting close means listening to the words and sharing the pain of the echo.

Do you take everything too personally? It will be some
relief for you to know that you are not the center of
the universe. When people are abrupt with you, unfair, unkind, unthinking—just generally unanything
supportive and pleasant—do you always get upset,
angry, and hurt? Such reactions are reasonable and
appropriate if their intention was to pick on you on
purpose. More often than not, they are pursuing some
other end, and are mostly unconscious of the impact
on you. For instance, they might just be blowing off

steam, reasserting their own power, boosting their own ego, taking care of some other imperative business. You might not even have entered their consciousness at all. In some cases, they may be unaware, rude, insensitive, self-centered, and callous, but look at who is getting devastated by it—YOU! Take yourself out of the center. Contemplate some other motives for their behavior, and perhaps you can exchange your personal suffering for solicitousness of them.

Is it hard for you to accept love when you're down? When you've experienced a failure, disappointment, or blow to your self-esteem, do you become an ornery critter if someone close tries to be solicitous? They had nothing to do with the problem, yet they are getting screamed at and abused for trying to be caring. You probably hate yourself for doing that, but it happens anyway. Why? First of all, you probably can't strike back at the true cause of your pain for lack of opportunity or fear of further reprisal. A loved one may seem like a safer reservoir for your pain-induced anger. Second, it may be humiliating for you to conceive of someone's seeing you at your worst. Your display of anger may be your reaction to your loved one's witnessing your narcissistic apocalypse. Third, you may be so frustrated and helpless that you become enraged because your loved one can't rescue you, kiss the "boo-boo," and make it all better. Let your loved one know what you're really feeling in all the complexity I've described. I think it'll help you feel better.

I don't like practical jokes or jokers. Practical jokes are not funny. When someone tells you bad news, waits for the depth of your emotional reaction, and then says, "Only kidding," that's not funny. When someone takes something that gives you pleasure and disturbs or distorts it in some way, that's not funny. In general, the end result of a practical joke is that someone is hurt, upset, or embarrassed. That's not funny. Then why are so many of you practical jokers? A practical joke is a way to dominate, to show your power or superiority, when because of your age, abilities, emotional immaturity, or lack of security you don't feel very powerful. In this case, the practical joke is generally aimed at someone you see as special. Envy and arrogance expressed sadistically through a practical joke cannot be salvaged by saying, "But it was only a joke." Keep in mind that there is a difference between a cute surprise which excites and a practical joke which demeans and causes pain. By the way, I'm not kidding.

Let's talk about saving face. I overheard a conversation between a mother and her little ten-year-old daughter who'd had a fight with her best friend. The mother said, "Why don't you call her up and apologize and tell her you want her to make up?" The little girl said, "I couldn't do that. She did wrong, too. I don't want to be the one to give in, and what if she doesn't want to make up?" The mother said, "Well, at least you'd know you'd been the bigger person." The little girl said, "So what? She won't see it that way." The mother said, "But you'll know." The little girl said, "No way. Let her come to me. Everybody will know that." The mother sighed and gave up. The little girl scowled and stalked off. I know the little girl is only ten, yet haven't you handled some of your relationships the same way, with appearance and scored points more important than what's right or fair or even healing. More relationships go by the wayside in just this way: pride and saving face before the warmth of continued friendship.

When should you butt your nose into someone else's business? It's too easy to look at the available information of someone else's situation and feel certain that your perspective or understanding is vital to him. Keep in mind that the information you have is never enough. Decisions are not made solely by the weight of the evidence. There is that mysterious factor of the emotional weight of that information. An observer can never assess what things mean to someone experiencing them. You can look at the obvious, the rational. The person in the situation lives the subtle, the irrational. Their conversations with you might help them better balance the rational and the emotional and help you appreciate the power of the emotional in their decision making. Butt your nose in as a sounding board and a support, not as a judge, critic, or expert. Butt your nose in without the demand that its directional signals be followed. Butt your nose in with love, or keep your nose to yourself.

Do you treat people as people, or as jobs you need them to do? You've got things to get done. You're intense, distracted, in a hurry. You bark orders, make demands, and you complain about a lack of ingenuity in others. It's possible their lack of motivation and effort is more a function of you than of their character. How? You are probably treating the people around you at work, in stores, and even at home as though they owed you some task. "If someone takes on a job or other responsibility," you say, "then they should take care of business without being milked." People are sensitive creatures and respond better to being treated like a person, a special person. Want to get more out of your people? Prime them with specialized attention. Ask about their family, vacation, new hairdo, suit of clothes, health, or hobbies. Any display of personal attention will make them feel less used and more useful. Deal with something off business before you get to something on business, and you will find that the person in them responds better to the person in you.

How can you go about learning how to trust? Many of you avoid personal closeness for fear of getting hurt again. The price may be long stretches of loneliness. You now want to have some personal companionship, warmth, and closeness, but how do you go about trusting again? One way might be just to decide to trust people, open up, be vulnerable, take your chances, and learn to deal with disappointment and hurt as facts of life. Disappointment and hurt *are* facts of life, and you need to see them as such, rather than as your personal fate. Yet deciding to trust people is similar to deciding not to trust people. It's an all-or-nothing decision. Learning to trust closeness in your life again is a specific event. Each person you choose to interact with is not a representative of the "them" who might hurt you. Each person is just that—a person. I'm not here to prove to you that people are trustworthy. I'm simply here with you to be me. Explore that concept for yourself.

What would it be like for you to go belly-up? If you've
had lots of experience with animals, been to a zoo, or
watched nature shows on TV, you've seen how most
animals fight. For the most part, it's ritualistic.
Individuals are rarely hurt significantly. The battles
end the moment one of them realizes it's one down,
and it goes belly-up. That's the signal that ends hostil-
ities. There is something to be learned here. Too many
times, the skirmishes you get into escalate past all
reason, compassion, and usefulness and your real personal choice. It's just that the tempers are up, and defending your turf, be it an idea, feeling, or statement,
becomes primary. As battles are won, the peace and
well-being of the relationship is often lost. What would
it be like for you to go belly-up—to give up battling,
whether you're right or wrong? Going belly-up means
a winner is not decided. The battle is abandoned.
Personal feelings, the significance of the relationship,
are attended to. It may seem like a loss in your mind.
Do it and you'll really experience what it can mean between friends.

Do you worry about being different? The curious
thing about your worries about being different is the

inherent belief that everyone else is the same. The pain of that position is that it ends up feeling like it's you against them. The truth is that the "they" are a whole bunch of "yous" who feel different, too. They just feel it about different things—race, religion, appearance, abilities, experience, background, thoughts, feelings, needs. I don't think it's the differentness, per se, that bothers you. It's that you value-judge differences as being somehow bad, which makes you bad. Therefore, you retreat into the wilderness of your pain, withdrawn and alone. An interesting tactic for you to try, should you want to escape from this inner hell, is to take an expedition into the differentness of someone else. Find out what it means, how it feels to him. You are all different in some special way. So often it's your attitude toward that difference that makes the difference between self-acceptance and socialization and withdrawal into that lonely wilderness of inner fear.

Are you pleasant now, pouty later? Are you honest about your hurt or needs at the time you feel them? Do you hide your feelings or pout in a gentle attempt to get taken care of? One woman came into therapy complaining bitterly about her husband's behavior and refusal to change. I watched them interact over many hours and observed that all of her so-called direct communications to him were either vague or about past unpleasant events. He was helpless to deal with the generalizations, and his apologies or explanations for the past events just fanned the fires. I worked on getting her to speak in the present. She became terribly upset and then silent. Dealing in the here and now is often perceived as threatening. It means exposing your immediate feelings, thoughts, and needs to observation and judgment. It means not having control. It sometimes means having to see yourself through other people's sensitivities. It means a lot that you might be avoiding. Give your partner a chance to give you what you want, and give yourself a chance to get what you need. Say what you're feeling and thinking at the time they happen.

When someone's upset, do you try to make her feel all better? When someone close to you expresses emotional pain, do you respond reflexively with, "Oh, it's not so bad," or, "It'll be okay," or, "Don't feel bad; it's really not that important"? I know you're trying to help. When you care about someone so much, you don't want her to be in pain. It may make you uncomfortable to deal with such strong emotions or to feel helpless to change things— in which case, your "make it all better" technique is really for your benefit more than hers. So when you try to make people feel better, you discount the validity of their feelings. They're saying they feel bad. You're saying it's silly or they shouldn't. The truth is that they feel what they feel. Maybe they need the time to mourn or face new painful realities. If you really want to be of help, listen, touch, and tell them you care.

"It's none of my business, but . . ." "I don't want to hurt you, but . . ." You don't, huh? Why is it that when it's none of your business, you butt in? Why is it that when you don't want to hurt, you do? Part of the explanation could be your need to be superior, expert, omniscient—all at the expense of the person you're trying to help. You, in fact, are taking advantage of his vulnerable position to finally ascend, to seem wise or important. No, this doesn't necessarily mean you don't care for him. Nor does it mean that you're a meanie. It could mean that you're not aware of your tendency to envy. Envy makes it all too easy to take advantage of an opportunity to be one up, if just for a moment. It's not that what you have to say isn't valid or sensible. But valid and sensible may not be very helpful at some of those emotional moments. Sometimes the best thing you can do with your lips is button them.

I'm going to say something to you, and I want you to remember your immediate reaction. Here goes: "Why don't you ever hug me anymore?" Did you feel instantly motivated to give me a hug, or a punch in the nose? Suppose I said instead, "Oh my, I've been feeling a bit grim today. I could use a hug from you now." Now do you feel more like giving me a hug? Why try to get something by complaining? Probably because you're frightened to death to get rejected. Your feisty, complaining stance is a show of strength, even lack of need. It's for your own protection. The tragedy is, you could protect yourself right out of any love or affection. From the experience you just had with me, you should know better from now on. Ask; don't manipulate. Risk showing need.

Are there times when your mouth seems to be on automatic pilot, saying the meanest, stupidest, cruelest, dumbest things you could ever imagine saying? You know you're wrong. You want to stop your mouth, but it just keeps going. What do you wish for at those moments? Right: someone to help you save face, help you stop your mouth with honor. Ever think that you could do the same for your beloved? Or is it more important for you to be hurt and angry so that you are justified in sticking it to them in some way, at some time? Helping each other save face during arguments that get messy and dirty is the most loving way to fight. Instead of retaliating one nasty comment for another, offer understanding, a hug, compassion. Time out. In other words, a way out. Only childish defensiveness can stop you from turning a fight into a touching moment of love and understanding.

Let's make apologizing a more selfish act. You may hesitate to apologize because you don't want to look weak, vulnerable, or one down, to be at anybody's mercy, lose face, or—ugh—look wrong. Now all those reactions have to do with how you think you'd feel with respect to someone else. It's time to be selfish. If you apologize for something you are wrong about, people will like and respect you more. If you apologize about something you're a little wrong about, you help the other person get in the mood to apologize to you. You like that, don't you? If you apologize about something you're not wrong at all about in your own mind, but it means something to the other person, then he'll probably do something nice for you, and you like that, don't you? If you apologize when you think you ought to get a weight off your back, then that feels better. All in all, apologizing may make you feel *really* good, so be selfish! Apologize more often.

Are you too suspicious? Are you always looking into, under, around, and through things people do and say to you, trying to find that ulterior motive, the real reason they were so nice? I'll bet you try to explain yourself by saying, "Lots of people are crummy and do or say things for other than the nicest motivations." I'll bet that some of the time, you're right. I'll also bet that you'd say, "This way, I won't get disappointment. Thinking they mean well, then finding out they don't. That hurts." And you know, you're right again. It's just that when you always have your defensive shields up you suffer all of the time, instead of just when your judgment was wrong and you took a direct hit in the gut. What's the point, though, of suffering all of the time to defend yourself against those few times when the worst does happen? If you doubt your ability to survive hurt, don't. With the continual emotional price you've been paying, you obviously can survive hurt.

Do you have good intentions and get blasted anyway? A couple I was counseling had a furious fight on the way in for their session. She had forgotten her appointment book at home and was terribly upset. He asked, "Is there anything important in it?" That's all she needed to hear. She said his comment was critical, demeaning; it just made things worse. He said he asked that because if it were important, he'd go back and get it for her. He then felt hurt that his intentions, never verbalized by the way, didn't protect him from the attack. Look, no matter how many self-help books you read on how to argue, communicate, and get along, you've got to use some common and loving sense. When your partner is upset, assume that she is going to be more sensitive than usual and not be totally able to follow Fight Rule 11(b) really well. However, since *you* are not upset, you can follow my Rule No. 1: When your partner is very upset, questions are often more upsetting. So why not lovingly make a generous and gentle offer? Or just go do it quietly and lovingly?

What's the real difference between an excuse and an explanation? "Don't give me your excuses. I don't want to hear it. You're just being defensive." While you're being yelled at like that, you're furiously thinking about how to say, "No, I'm just trying to explain what happened," without sounding defensive. Can't be done. So now you start screaming, too. You could split hairs about the fine difference between excusing and defending and you'd still be off the track. You see, what they are really saying is, "I feel hurt by what you've done regardless of the reason you did it. And you are only attending to your own guilt and not caring about me and how I feel." So any kind of discussion centered on your deed or your motive won't be satisfactory until you've first acknowledged the other person's predicament, pain, and disappointment. And I mean acknowledged it with sincerity. Then you can take the time and clarify.

Can anything good come of complaining? Complaining is important to your relationship. Without it, you'd be isolated and unfulfilled. You might think that avoiding conflict builds closeness. No. Avoiding mean and vicious conflict is important, but you need conflict resolution to bring closeness. When you and your beloved come to each other with unique experiences, expectations, and fantasies, they won't be appreciated or fulfilled without you both verbalizing and bouncing your feelings and ideas back and forth. Hoping you'll be understood and taken care of in a special way is dangerous. Hoping is a secret experience and one that too often promises disappointment simply because your partner is not clairvoyant. Closeness comes from clarifying and working through differences. There's no magical special person who matches up perfectly in advance. That's a deadly, romantic notion which robs from you the joy and satisfaction of growing to know someone.

Do you give up on friends too easily? When you meet someone you seem to hit it off with immediately, do you dive right into feelings of deep friendship? Are those feelings too quickly demolished by other feelings of disappointment or betrayal? Making and having friends is tricky business. The expectations and behaviors are very different from those for family or lovers or spouses. The ties are not based on blood, sex, or legalities. Probably the strongest tie of friendship is pure and simple acceptance. You don't have to agree on everything, share everything, or even know everything. Let your friends have the quirky parts of them that don't meet your tastes or expectations. You don't have to take them on yourself, you know. Don't write off friends too quickly. In your haste to judge and dismiss, you might find yourself alone more often than you'd like to be. Think about concessions people in your life have made in order to keep you in theirs.

Are you terrified to admit you've done something wrong? What's your style of avoiding taking the rap when you've earned it? Do you deny all knowledge of what's going on? Do you list extenuating circumstances? Do you blame someone else? The bottom line is that people get angry and tired of your excuses, and you've got to expend time and energy continually supporting your shaky position. Underneath it all, you probably worry that if you admit to being wrong, people will hate you and abandon you. Keep up trying to always look right and you may get that anyway. Try this exercise: For one whole week, find things you've goofed up on—anything from scrambling eggshell pieces into the eggs to forgetting to take the mortgage check in on time. Announce to each and all every mistake or wrongdoing, intentional or not. Have the experience of voluntarily getting it all off your chest. See how you feel. See how everyone reacts to you.

Maybe you're being just a little too sensitive. If, more often than not, someone's mood or tone deeply upsets you, if a criticism or complaint of even a minor nature is enough to seriously set you back, if you are always interpreting and second-guessing everyone else's motives or intent, perhaps you're being too sensitive. We think of the sensitivity of creative people, psychics, and those in the helping professions as central to their functioning. It then becomes an antenna which facilitates expression and communication. Your oversensitivity may already have proved itself to be exhausting, distorting, and destructive. How can there be open communication if you are already certain you know what's going on and why? How can there be any sensitivity to the other person's feelings and needs if you're always so sure everything only has to do with you? Next time you feel your feelings twinged by someone else's word or deed, ask him how he's feeling.

What's a good way to handle criticism? Criticism hurts, constructive or not. It's not pleasant to have people point out your deficiencies, shortcomings, and blemishes. So what do you do? Get all defensive and criticize them back? Tell them, "Who cares, kiss off"? Or do you eat it and stew? Does any of that make you feel better? My suggestion about handling criticism is the same whether or not the criticism is friendly or justified. When someone wants to offer you criticism, seem interested, curious. Ask questions. Ask for clarification; ask for examples. Once you put yourself in the position of asking for more information, you become stronger in your own eyes and theirs. The conversation might turn out to have some useful information for you. You might come out of it as friends. And if that isn't desired, you still will come out of it respected.

Let's hear it for generalizations! Generalizations can be fun. You get to sound knowledgeable, definite, profound, even powerful. And you always have an edge. When people argue with you, all you have to do is seem to give an inch. "Well, okay—*almost* everybody." And you really haven't given anything. Take this generalization: Generally, the generalizations you make about others reflect more about you than they tell us anything objective about others. Here's a typical example. "All people will use you if you give them a chance." Now, assuming my generalization, that reflects more about you than the "them" it indicates. It could mean that you feel fearful and helpless about revealing your needs and asking for what you want. So you end up doing the other person's will and feeling resentful afterwards. Or it could mean that you over-give as a hint that you want something. Of course, this is only true sometimes, for some of you—generally speaking.

Are you shy? Do you think you are the only one in the world who feels shy? Shyness is a universal experience. We all worry to some extent about how others see and judge us. We all express it differently. Some of us retreat into thin air. Others put on a happy face. Some hide it behind alcohol, drugs, and negativism. The point is, we are all basically isolated creatures, wrapped up by this skin envelope in a container called the body. Shyness is a matter of turning your eyeballs inward, seeing only the isolation within. To bridge shyness, to make contact, we all have to turn those eyeballs around and literally take the sight and experience of others within. We do that with the tools of interest, tolerance, compassion, and communication. It is not half the people's responsibility to make contact with the other half. It's a responsibility and pleasure we all have.

Is it hard for you to kiss and make up? Would making up be more palatable to you if the other person gave in first? Think of it. The other says, "Okay, I'm sorry. Let's forget it, all right?" And then you, in your magnanimity, say, "Well, all right." Great scene, with you keeping the power. Feels great, doesn't it? Feels like you haven't lost anything. Nor have you given anything. If making up and giving in are the same to you, then you probably don't truly resolve problems between you and others. You probably make others decide that they must bend or lose you. Keep going like this, and losing you might seem more attractive to them in time. What's more important to you? The regard, affection, and involvement of others, or the ego gratification of winning? Someone taught you all too well and painfully what it was like to be on the losing end. Now you're teaching others. Instead, show them humanity.

Fear is an interesting thing. Fear has such power in your lives. You're scared to meet people because they might not like you. You're scared to try something new because you might fail. You're scared about being open because—well, you're sometimes not quite sure what you're scared of. Fear is anything you make it. When I was a kid, my parents took me to see a scary movie about a dinosaur that attacked New York City. It ate people and taxicabs, leveled buildings, and squashed everything. When we came home, I couldn't go to bed until my mom looked under the bed and in the closet, just in case the dinosaur picked my room to hide out in. Now some dinosaurs were actually vegetarian, and certainly too tall to hide under the bed! It didn't matter. I was scared. Lucky for me, I had my mom help me scout out my fear, and then I could go to sleep. Too many times you keep your fears fed by not expressing them and exploring them with someone you trust, someone who cares about you. You'll live freer and sleep better if you do.

# CHAPTER 4

# *Personal Responsibility*

What do you really mean when you say, "You're right, it's my fault"? There are several meanings possible when you admit to responsibility. Most of them are evasive. For example, you may admit to responsibility to be sarcastic, that's usually obvious from the tone. Or your admission could be the way you stop the discussion—how can you argue with a person who says, "You're right. I'm bad"? Another motivation is to get the heat off you. Once you admit to how bad you are, your partner usually feels obligated to say, "Well, it's okay, it's not so bad, really." It seems that much of the time you admit to fault, guilt, or responsibility, you don't mean it. It's not difficult to prove this. Think about the last time you admitted guilt. Did you become defensive when your partner went into specifics? If you did, then you can be certain that when you agreed in general to responsibility, you had little intention of facing specific truths.

What does it mean to be loyal? To some of you, loyalty means you'll follow along with someone right or wrong. That's uncomplicated, but dangerous. It means you could get into painful predicaments and that your friend has a blind shadow, rather than a safe, responsive sounding board. Sticking by someone does not mean following; it means being caring and concerned enough to be honest and open with your ideas and feelings. It means being supportive of that person, if not his acts. You parents struggle with that when your children begin to live by rules other than yours. You love and want your children, so you separate them from their acts, as they must separate you from yours. Loyalty is not blind; it is aware and tolerant. Blind loyalty is mimicry for the sake of security. It has no wisdom or compassion, both of which are desperately needed by all of us. Therefore, in giving loyalty, you do not give up yourself, you give of yourself.

Whatever happened to your New Year's resolutions? Remember your resolutions list? No? Well, I'm not surprised. Who wants to remember a list of how crummy you are and what you have to do to be salvaged? Your list was probably too long, the resolutions too huge, and the rewards too minimal to maintain any of your enthusiasm. The rewards need to be built into your resolutions for change. The rewards need to be concrete rather than philosophical. One of the ways I got myself comfortable about facing scary things like an exam was to promise myself something I loved upon completion. Then I would focus in on that reward whenever I started to get uptight about the thing I had to do. It gave me perspective, made me realize that there was something beyond that fearful task, and I was being good to myself. Try facing your most difficult assignments with a tangible reward of your own choosing as a promise. You might find the tasks become more appealing.

Do you worry about being lazy? Is it unbearably difficult for you to kick back, relax, play games, do nothing, when you know there's some work that needs to be done? Do you feel guilty having fun because a little voice in your head berates you for not taking care of responsibilities? Those feelings often have unpleasant behaviors attached to them, like when you monitor and criticize others for their lack of motivation and responsibility because they rest, or when you put others second to your work and accuse them of interference or undermining you. Sound familiar? If so, you're not living your life. You're sacrificing yourself at the altar of a tyrannical memory—a memory of a childhood time when you tried so hard to get love, approval, and acceptance from someone who seemed so hard to please, so hard to reach. You're still trying to work hard enough to be okay, and you never stop trying because the only one left with the power to tell you you're okay is you, and you're not listening.

Are you a creature of bad habits? Now, why don't you drink, eat, and smoke less? Exercise, play, and read more? I'll bet you're getting ready to say, "Oh yeah, I know I should do that. I'll look into it." Well, don't bother. That's a stall anyway. Bad habits have a lot to do with self-indulgence in the shadow of low self-esteem. Those naughty pleasures soothe you in ways you are loath to give up. Yes, eating too much is bad for you. You know that. But doesn't it feel good when you're doing it? Better than having to sit with feelings of anxiety, discomfort, loneliness, and despair? Bad habits are a Band-Aid therapy, effective but temporary. Bad habits are also a means of rebellion—you are showing that you can do whatever, whenever, and however you want, no matter what anyone else thinks or wants. You'll show 'em. If you really want to break bad habits, you first need to clarify their deeper meaning. If you are hurting emotionally, it's time to face that. If you're forty-five and still battling with your parents, your spouse, and your children over a sense of importance, it's time to face that. Bad habits survive on bad feelings inside you.

Are you ever satisfied with yourself? Do you take up one job, start feeling good about what you're accomplishing, then get antsy and start something else? Do you begin to get excited about finishing a project well, then start finding fault with it or feel let down when you're done? Do you ever have the sensation of recognizing and enjoying a job well done? Your childhood should have allowed you experiences of feeling satisfied with yourself based on the sincerity if not the quality of your efforts. Instead, you heard, "Never stop and rest on your laurels," or, "You're only as good as your next job," or, "You finished it? What took you so long? And what's wrong with that part over there?" Then I can understand your inability to enjoy the process and the accomplishment. That would give you a constant trickle of dread and resentment. How to get out of this trap? Do some things you enjoy privately, and only for the time span in which you get a kick out of it; and reward yourself all along the way.

Have you thought about making a major change in your life lately? You may be a career woman over thirty-five recently deciding to have a baby. You may be a professional man over forty now contemplating an entire change in lifestyle. You might be at home deciding to get a college diploma. Whoever and whatever, stop for a moment and ask yourself whether you're wanting to add a dimension to your life or hoping to alleviate pain from your life. It makes a difference. If you're hoping that having a child, new job or lifestyle, or diploma is going to give you all the happiness you've been missing or repair damage, you're going to be painfully disappointed. All of those opportunities require much from you immediately while giving returns mostly down the line. A baby can't repair your disappointing childhood or your present marriage. A diploma can't fix your fractured sense of personal worth and well-being. A new job can't fix your frustrations or unhappy relationships. These changes are not cures. They are added dimensions.

Do you blame all bad things on someone else? You shouldn't underestimate yourself so much. You must give yourself credit for being able to mess up, be mean, fail, stumble, or be wrong just like anyone else. Who told you that you weren't allowed to have those qualities in your repertoire of humanness? You should chastise them for disallowing you to run on all cylinders. Seem silly of me, maybe even sarcastic? I mean it. If you're not allowed to be all the parts of you, then you're not allowed to be your true self. How can you ever really feel loved or worthy of love if you must deny the existence of some of you? If you must struggle to hide parts of yourself by making others responsible for them, then deep down inside you must know that means you *as you* are unacceptable. That's a painful awareness. Imagine being loved in spite of and with your "naughties." Imagine someone standing by you while you work through those "naughties." Imagine the freedom of growth and change instead of hiding and blaming. The next time you do something wrong, take full credit for it with pride. Work it through. It's your right.

Are you fed up? Are you sick and tired, frustrated, angry, upset, and generally disgusted with the slice of life served to you? It's easy to feel this way since life, like a cake, doesn't have cherries all the way through it. So what do you need to do? Abandon hope and dreams? Give up on your needs? No. You must decide what your true, deep needs, hopes, and dreams are. Maybe you need to feel accomplished, have some fun, relax, meet a challenge, have a success, feel important, needed, or necessary. Whatever it is, it's up to you to find some ways to create those for yourself without leaving it up to fate or other people. One actor friend of mine was feeling like a failure. In his frustration, he wouldn't allow any time for anything else. Finally, on a skiing trip, he experienced success feelings, making it down a slope in one unbroken piece. Don't wait for it; go out and get it.

Do you make too many assumptions? I love the word "assumption." I'm reminded of one teacher who said, "Beware of your assumptions lest you make the first three letters of that word out of yourself." Sometimes you make assumptions so you don't have to take the time to check things out. Checking it out might bring up information that could get in the way of what you want and are going to do. Sometimes you make assumptions as a means of second-guessing someone, as a kind of ballet around his objections or displeasure. Sometimes you make assumptions because you're stuck in one mode of thinking about things, as though it were the only mode possible. Sometimes you make assumptions because it allows you to seem knowledgeable and in control, on top of things. Assumptions aren't really bad things. They can be a first step you make in planning or understanding a situation. Yet they are only as good as the effort you put in to validate them. Make your assumptions commas in your paragraphs of life, not periods.

What's a good way to wait? The first thing to remember about waiting is that it has no power. Waiting doesn't mean your anticipated package will be delivered. If you generally fly into rages when your waiting doesn't pay off, you've forgotten this number-one rule. The second thing to remember about waiting is that it is not a trance. A trance is simply focused attention. If your waiting means emotional, intellectual, and behavioral suspended animation, you must remember that you are not in the twilight zone. Time is continuing. Experiences and opportunities are passing, not waiting for you. The third thing to remember about waiting is that it is a risk, so make it a calculated risk. An investment of time, effort, patience, and direction generally means that other options are being excluded for the time being. It's like playing Monopoly—sometimes holding on to some property becomes more of a liability than a good investment. So set up some parameters of time and circumstance rather than leaving your waiting open-ended.

Are you fighting someone else for possession of your identity? Adolescents often feel they have to fight their parents, teachers, and other authority figures for their identity. They get identity and power all mixed up, something maturity is supposed to clear up. Yet you as adults have accused others of trying to obliterate, steal, or manipulate your identity because you felt weak or frightened, as well as needy of their power. If you've been hesitant to assert yourself, think for yourself, defend yourself, inquire or require, then you gave up creating your own singular identity. Instead, you created an image you hoped would be universally accepted, liked, unattacked. If you chose to go down the rapids on a raft without a paddle, is it fair to blame the current for pushing you around? No one owns your identity, your personhood. It is defined within you and evidenced by your interactions with others. Yelling at others to give you space or your own mind is to prove you have abdicated your own.

Do you set a hectic schedule for yourself? A couple I was working with were one month away from having their first baby. They had started out in a natural childbirth program together where the father learns to be a coach in the delivery room as the wife gives birth without anesthetic. At first he attended the classes with her and went through the daily exercise routine. As time went on, it seemed that his work requirements, paddle tennis tournaments, meetings, therapy, and, of course, need for rest got in the way of his par ticipating in the program. He regretted having such a hectic schedule that got in the way of the birthing exercises, but hectic schedules usually have a purpose other than the accidental piling up of things. Sometimes they keep you from feeling certain feelings. Sometimes they make you feel important and successful, or prove you're not lazy. For this couple, the husband's hectic schedule kept him from being involved in a birth he couldn't admit ambivalence about. It was as though avoiding it would make it go away. Your hectic schedule *does* mean something.

Do you let someone else call the shots for your life? Are you going with someone, not really knowing what he's thinking and feeling about you, but you're hoping? Are you going with someone, not really certain he'll ever make a commitment to you, but you're hoping? Your uncertainty and insecurity go on and on. It seems so bleak, yet you wonder, should you stay or leave? You just keep staying and hoping. If you were pollen, then your waiting around for the wind or an insect to carry you away would have a purpose—pollination. That means birth and growth. Plants were designed that way. People weren't. Your waiting is not in anticipation of living; it is an abdication of living. It is a fantasy which promises happiness only when you're holding on to someone else's ankles—and have you noticed, they are usually kicking to get free of the burden. It is your responsibility to direct and design your own life; then you'll be in the position to share it with someone willing and capable.

Are you still trying to find yourself? The notion of finding yourself implies that you've not yet been dis-covered or that you've been misplaced. That must mean that the present you is a temporary prototype waiting to be fully perfected, or a momentary fill-in, waiting for the return of the truly meaningful version. Both those notions are excuses, distortions, and at-tempted escapes from responsibility. If you are not your true and final self because you haven't quite got-ten there yet, or you've been detoured, then who can judge or demand of you? The truth is that at all times in your life, you are the total you. It might be that you don't feel adequate, acceptable, or at peace. It might be that you feel confused more often than not. It might be that your fears and others' powers have more control over you than you'd like. Whatever the disap-pointment or concern, that is you now. Your experi-ences, strengths, weaknesses, fears, needs, and deeds are your tools. Saying, "I'm not me, really" is to deny the truth of who you are and to lose grip of the tools you need to build your future.

Do you complain about your guardian devil? Guardian angels are supposed to save you from tight spots and desperate straits, all in your best interests. What's a guardian devil? Someone who saves you from tight spots and desperate straits, at times when it's *not* in your best interests. Guardian angels just happen. You pick your guardian devils. They are the spouses you complain about. You say, "Oh, I'd like to do that, but my guardian devil won't let me. They get angry. I wanted to learn to read or paint or study, but my guardian devil says it's silly." You complain about being bossed and mistreated. When asked why you don't just go and do the things anyway, you open your eyes wide and say, "Well, how could I? There'd be a fight, unhappiness." You pick a guardian devil, a no-giver to protect you from the things you're afraid of—creativity, autonomy, risk taking, and failure. You're off the hook—a poor, oppressed, long-suffering individual who lives on others' sympathies for your plight until they realize it's self-imposed. Don't nag at your guardian devils. They're protecting you just the way you want.

How many times do you defend yourself by saying, "I would have if *you...*" did or didn't do something. Very clever. Somehow, you've just made your partner responsible for your behavior. You're saying that your ability or willingness to do the right things is dependent upon what or how your spouse does or says something. Fascinating. Did you realize you were so easily manipulated into not being the kind of person you'd normally be? That's not what you intend, is it? In blaming the other person for your forgetfulness, unwillingness, or sloppiness, you're simply trying to take the heat off yourself by putting it on your loved one. You're not willing to own up to your feelings and the meanings of your actions. Your number-one priority is simply not to look like the one who is wrong, regardless of the price your partner and the relationship ends up paying. From now on, explain yourself with only "I" and "me" in your sentences. Struggle to leave out the words "if you." You'll get more understanding and love just the way you want it.

Are you not selfish enough? A lot of your problems might be solved better if you were more selfish. For instance, when someone you care about is not giving you all you need or want, do you withdraw or push her away? Do you take nothing because you can't have everything? Be more selfish! Don't punish yourself. Get from them what they can or will give. Do you feel yourself torn between spending all your time at work or spending all your time with your family, friends, and pets? Be more selfish! If work *and* family *and* friends *and* hobbies are all important for you, don't choose between them. Get as much of all of it as you can. Blend 'em, balance 'em, do whatever it takes to get all of what would give you pleasure and satisfaction in your life. You look at so much of what you need or would enjoy as an imposition on the time you need to spend on obligations and responsibilities. Be more selfish. You are not simply a mechanism of accomplishments. You are a person with needs and feelings. Be more selfish. Enjoy your life and the people in it.

Why should you have to do things you don't want to do? When you were a kid, your parents were always telling you to do things you didn't want to do, everything from cleaning your room, brushing your teeth, studying, dressing, behaving . . . you just knew that when you grew up and they couldn't boss you around anymore, you would never again do anything you didn't want to do. Here you are an adult in the very predicament you thought you'd left behind. You have to exercise, eat properly, fulfill responsibilities, deal with problems you'd rather ignore. Now you don't have a parent to remind you. Now you have your conscience, sense of responsibility, a boss, a spouse. You could become angry and continue your adolescent rebelliousness. You could become resigned and plod through it all numbly. You could work on making it fun by rewarding yourself in private little ways. It's important to remember that some of the things people do for *you,* things you depend on and enjoy, are often done in spite of their not really feeling like it.

Let's take a second look at guilt. You've seen all the psychology articles and experts working feverishly to exorcize the world of guilt as though it were only an inappropriate alien infestation. Boy, what a relief it's been, finding out that you don't have to feel responsible for anything or anyone and that guilt is nature's way of manipulating you! For those of you who are desperate to be loved, attached, and protected, that may be an appropriate issue. But for most of you, guilt may be a good emotional signal that something may be wrong, the way that pain is a physical signal that something may be wrong in your body. One man I was counseling was sometimes living with his wife, sometimes having sex with his wife, and always dating other women as part of his three-year quest for a divorce. He said one day that he would really like to help his wife move on with her life. When I suggested that moving in and out of her house, having sex with her when he needed it, probably wasn't helpful to her in that regard, he said, "You're making me feel guilty." And?

What's the difference between fault and responsibility? You may be in battles with your beloved over issues of who's at fault about something. What happens? You both get angry, hurt, defensive, generally bent all out of shape, simply because nobody wants to take the fault of the whole thing! Or you may be easily gotten to with guilt, in which case, if someone cleverly points out even one tiny little thing you did wrong, you're willing to go up the river for the whole predicament. There's a big, important difference between fault and responsibility. For instance, "It's your fault we're in this crummy restaurant." Now, it is your fault if you blindfolded, tied up, and hauled that person in against his will. If you haven't done that, then a suggestion or a request is not a fault, it's a contributing responsibility. Taking responsibility has to do with acknowledging your participation. Fault has you owning total responsibility for everyone. Make arguments about fault become discussions about responsibility.

You've got to stop acting like a flower waiting for a bee! Flowers create new life by waiting for an insect or the wind to transfer pollen to another flower. Are you building your life with the same precarious passivity?

Are you afraid to ask for what you want? Are you afraid to even want? Asking is not pushing. Refusing is not being mean. Wanting is not selfish. You may have your head filled with all sorts of frightening warnings, such as those handed down to you from someone who wanted total control, or modeled for you by someone afraid of taking control and the responsibilities that come with it. Without taking an active role in your life, no one can really know what you want, what to give you. You will probably never feel a sense of belonging because you haven't participated in establishing whatever you're in. Stop being invisible. Start being involved. You can begin this simply by letting people around you know your thoughts, feelings, and ideas and by giving them a chance to adapt to the new you.

"I didn't realize I caused you all this trouble." "If I'm such a burden to you, I'll just go away and not talk to you about this anymore." If you've been on the receiving end of that, you already know how it feels: infuriating, guilt-provoking, frustrating. You feel trapped into trying to be more helpful than is reasonable. Then the resentment begins. If you've *delivered* that sentiment, then you know how you feel: helpless, frightened, and angry. And in defensiveness, you threaten withdrawal or even suicide as an attempt to make sure you won't be criticized or rejected. You might start believing your own press and precipitate your own aloneness or toy with your own death. You, the receiver, must set reasonable limits to what you will do and what you can and will accept as your responsibility, and you must accept that the threat might happen. You, the threatener, may need some help to find less destructive ways of gaining attention, control, love, and caretaking.

Are enthusiasm and patience only memories to you? Are you often tired and bored? We all have days like that; that's to be expected. But if you can barely remember not feeling that way, you're burned out. You might have tried drinking or drugs to stop the feelings. You might have abused your family, blaming them for your pain. You might have quit, dropped out, become callous or cynical. You can't just pick around for one simple explanation for burnout and try to fix or eliminate it. You're burned out because your cup ran over with all that is going on in your life. You have expectations of yourself at work, at home, with relatives, in your community, and so on. Write down each one of your responsibilities and listen to yourself justify the why and how you take it on. Are you forcing yourself because of guilts or fears? Then those are the enemies. Get your life back and get more out of your life by making sure that you operate out of your will, and not your guilt.

Remember when you were a child and there was no such thing as exercise? Biking, running, playing ball, and skating were routine in your life. It was called "playing." What kind of play do you have in your life now? Movies, cards, TV? And weekend tennis frenzies? Maybe. You know you need exercise for your waistline, your heart, and your disposition. So you join the health club. You buy all the proper shoes and clothes with color-coordinated sweatbands. You go regularly at first, and then come the excuses and the rain checks to yourself. In your childhood, physical activity was a natural part of your day, of your life. Now you have responsibilities, and less energy. And you have rules that play comes after the work is done, whenever that is. Let's not forget that exercise hurts and it just chews up your time. How sad and unhealthy it is that some of your childhood attitudes are lost when you grow up. What will it take for you to come out and play?

What do you think it means to cope? I read and answer your letters individually. You impress me, move me, and tickle me. Sometimes you stump me. Like when you ask about how to cope, when you're really asking me how to make an uncomfortable situation go away, not exist, not touch you anymore. I'm thinking in particular of one of your letters about caring for an aged parent. The letter asked more about how to rid yourself of the responsibility of caring for that parent and the guilt for giving up that responsibility. That's not coping; that's abdicating. Caring for an aged and infirm parent can bring anger, frustration, despair, loneliness. Doing the best you can, getting support for yourself so that you can do the best you can—that's coping. So, if there isn't a self-help group in your area, start one. Get the help you need to cope with the complex emotional difficulties involved. Coping doesn't mean finding a way to force life to change; it means adapting to what is.

Is it hard for you to treat yourself because you're always left wondering whether or not you should have? Do you really deserve it? That's left over from your childhood. When you were a kid and asked for something, did your folks say, "Well, okay. But were you a good little boy?" Or, "If you're a good little girl, we'll get you that"? When you were a child, there was an authority figure to make the assessment of your worthiness and to bestow upon you the goodies which you earned. Then there was relief in the getting. But now that you have to be your *own* parent and child, do you have trouble deciding whether or not you're worthy, lovable, or entitled? The big question of your adult years is, are you willing to take the responsibility and the consequences of your actions? Maybe that's how you ought to measure your earning power and not by performing and holding out your hat.

How can you get out of feeling crummy? You're probably thinking that what you have to do is wait to feel better before you can start doing some fun or nice things for yourself. The truth is that the wait prolongs your misery. It might just help you to do some things for yourself and then watch your spirits rise, even if it's only for the duration of the distraction. Just as feeling crummy triggers a kind of negative thinking which feeds into its own misery, feeling better does the same. Be careful that you're not holding on to feeling miserable just so that you can get out of certain responsibilities or so that you can accumulate what you feel is long-overdue attention or sympathy. That might work for the short run, then you're going to find others running out of patience and interest. I'll admit, a bit of wound licking may give you the time you need to rest, to regain perspective and motivation. Then give yourself a break. Treat yourself well in spite of everything, even yourself.

So you eat all kinds of junk food and you get all sick and nervous? Maybe you can remember being emotionally reimbursed with junk food by your mom or dad who was trying to make you feel better. What might have been more useful was help in learning that you could survive disappointment and failure. Or that problems were there to be solved, not to be dissolved. If food was the currency of love or repair when you were a child, it's all too natural for you now, as an adult, to hang on to the old ways. Remember, though, that this kind of eating is addictive behavior, in the same sense as drugs or alcohol or spending money. You feel the pain, think you can't tolerate the frustration, and you resort to an immediate high, immediate satisfaction. You know you're not becoming stronger but weaker, as you persistently reinforce an inner belief that you can't make it any other way. A diet is not enough. You need to get support to build new skills for survival and conquest instead of survival by default.

Is anything truly hopeless? I counsel many people who wonder whether or not they should give up in some situation where they've tried what they feel is everything. Will he ever stop drinking? Will the tension at work ever ease up? Will my mother ever stop criticizing me? Of course, there's no way for me to predict the future, so what do you do? Some people will tell you to hang in there forever, just in case it does change, or you'll be sorry! Some people will tell you to drop it and run, or you'll be sorry! Only you know what you can tolerate, how much you've already invested, how much return you got for that investment, and how much more you're willing to invest. That may sound mechanical. Yet real life has its limits and people their limitations. If continuing gives you mostly pain or leaving gives you mostly guilt, perhaps some personal support and professional intervention might help. You don't need to lose hope. You may need to transfer it to a more willing location.

Are you the one who reminds your friends and relatives about how much more grown-up they should be? Do you feel weighted down being the one who takes care of most responsibilities? You're in a bind inside yourself. One part of you feels compelled and proud to be grown-up and competent. Another part of you, hidden, wants to be free and taken care of. This part of yourself scares you, and what scares you, you deny and even punish in yourself and in others. That's where your nagging and criticizing of others comes from. Maybe you've had too much responsibility as a child. Maybe you've always had to take care of yourself, and now you're afraid to be dependent, afraid to relax your control and vigilance. Change, but take it slowly. Treat yourself to luxuries, happy quiet moments, and most importantly, start sharing your true feelings and fears with loved ones.

Why do you have time for some things, but not others? Oh yeah, I know it doesn't really mean anything that you were able to work overtime last week but couldn't get around to doing that favor or even having some fun. Uh huh. Sure it doesn't. Let's be honest for a fraction of a second. You do the things you choose to do over doing things that are demanded of you, threaten you, overly challenge you, or don't contribute to how you'd like to see yourself. Not having time becomes your disguised means of fighting back against someone else's potential control over you, or hiding from some conflict. I'm not saying that you shouldn't have the right to choose how you want to invest your efforts. When you are using excuses such as not having the time, you are giving up free choice and giving in to your fears and discomforts. Through excuses, you are avoiding learning about yourself, not allowing yourself to adapt or really be close to anyone. The game is always in the way.

"Well, I'd be home more if you wouldn't be so frumpy around the house!" "Oh yeah? I'd fix myself up more if you would be more romantic." Oh my. Ever been in that kind of round robin of blame where each of you holds the other responsible for your behavior? Think of it this way. If someone else is responsible for causing behaviors you don't like in yourself, why do you let them manipulate you into being the kind of person you don't want to be? Are you really a puppet? No, of course not. What you are is a person who has fallen into the old trap of making someone else carry the blame for you, getting you off the hook. If it's someone else's fault, then there's no reason to look any deeper into yourself, is there? If you really wanted to give, you wouldn't let the other stop you. Don't let anyone keep you from being the person you want to be. If you want to be home on time, look nice, or be nice, do it! No "buts," please. If you don't want to be or do those things after all, look inside yourself for the reason.

Do you put all your emotional eggs in one basket? Is your whole identity and happiness wrapped up in only one aspect of your life? No matter how much you love parenting, work, or a relationship, relying totally on any one of these experiences for a sense of well-being is dangerous. Kids grow up and out, there are layoffs, demotions, firings; and a relationship changes or ends. These things happen as a natural part of life. Under the best of circumstances, you are deeply affected by these changes or crises. But if you don't have any other emotional or intellectual involvements to fall back on, you may fall over into a psychologically messy heap. You may put all your energies into one thing because you think that's the only way to do it right. Or because you're afraid to try new things. Whatever your reason, it's a trap, so get out of it. Get involved in more things. You'll have more to give. You'll have more security. Spread those emotional eggs around.

# CHAPTER 5

# *Self-esteem*

Is it really too late for you? Is it too late for you to start school? Tell the truth? Begin a fitness program? Become a writer? Pick up tennis? Love someone? Is that what you say, it's too late? Perhaps you're right, but only in part. It may be too late for you to train for Wimbledon, but it's not too late to learn tennis. It may be too late for you to win that person back into your life, but it's not too late to repair hurts. When you rely on lateness as an excuse, you avoid the deep texture of life. Humility, pain, poignancy, struggle, compromise, and challenge are all potentials for deeply gratifying experiences. One lady was afraid to go back to school at forty-three. Finally deciding to give it a try, she said, "I'm doing well and it surprises me. It scares me, but I love it. I'm surprised that I can be scared and still enjoy myself." Select one of five things you've been saying it's too late for you to begin. Do it, and you too may surprise yourself.

Are you scared to feel your own feelings? Do you run from feeling your own feelings? There are several ways you do this: by drinking or using drugs; by distracting yourself with excessive work, sports, or sexual encounters; and by doing whatever it takes to make the threatening situation go away. Your immediate awareness of those frightening feelings does go away, but they'll be back. Here's an example. Someone close to you isn't treating you well. You hint, you beat around the bush, but you never handle this problem directly. You say you don't want to upset them, but actually you're afraid of their anger and how that would make you feel, and since you're so afraid of what it might feel like, you avoid the situation. In doing this, you never find out what that feeling is really like, or whether you can learn to get through it or grow from it. I suggest you arrange a situation that forces you to experience your most feared feeling. You may surprise yourself with your own strength.

Why do you get so uncomfortable when someone or something is different? Something different arouses your interest. Sounds exciting? Hopefully. Makes you a bit uncomfortable; even anxious? Highly likely. Although boring, the known and familiar brings a warm sense of security. Remember your first "blankie"? The way you like your favorite sandwich made? Do you remember the burst of discomfort you had when a detour sign made you take a different route home? Or when Mommy married a new daddy? The unknown, exciting as it can be, brings challenges, new rules, new expectations. It literally forces you to increase your awareness, involvement, and risk taking. It was so much more comfortable when you could take everything for granted, wasn't it? That's why different scares you. That's why you defend yourself by judging it harshly and negatively. You do that in the hopes of making it disappear.

Are there things you would like to do but avoid doing because of how it might seem? Do you avoid sewing because you don't want to seem like an unliberated woman? Do you avoid needlepoint because other guys will call you a sissy? Do you avoid lifting weights because you don't want to be called unfeminine? Do you avoid cleaning and decorating your house for fear you will be labeled "henpecked"? That's the small child in you afraid of rejection for being different. That is a problem. The way you have chosen to solve it is by rejecting yourself so that you won't have to be rejected by others. That's leading your life as a sacrifice on the altar of others' whims. It is important to be liked and respected—not only by others, though, by yourself first. When you give yourself respect and pleasure, you have more to give to others. That's the real honey to attract caring friends with, isn't it?

Have you ever said, "Oh, I know I'd be just great at that if I wanted to." We all want to feel terrific at something. It's like having your name on some niche of existence. Being great at something is also a way to get some applause, praise, and approval. Now, that sounds pretty good, doesn't it? So why would you avoid all those goodies by talking about what you can do instead of doing it? Because you're afraid. In proclaiming your greatness without expended effort, you hope to give yourself the illusion of worth, even superiority. Trying anything would bring failure and the loss of your illusion, so you don't try. When you say, "I'd be just great at that, I know it, so I don't have to do it," it's similar to the emotional phenomenon of New Year's resolutions. Somehow by saying it, you're trying to convince yourself, it's done, done well, so no more need for guilt. This is a terrible trap. You never have the chance to experience conquests and successes. You exist like a fragile bubble of self-esteem, worried that someone or something will burst your illusions.

Are you too quick to give up? When you find there's something you don't know, can't find, can't figure out, can't do immediately, do you give up? If you do, you may say nasty things about the situation in order to explain the failure, yet you're still left with the pain of the failure and with feelings of frustration, the very feelings you tried to avoid by giving up. Failure and frustration are not fun experiences. They're difficult and unpleasant, at best. Something, though, makes them red stoplights, rather than yellow warning lights. Something makes you run from them rather than run through them. Punitive experiences you had as a child may have taught you all too painfully the dangers of trying, the safety of quitting. The price: your self-esteem. You can change. Start thinking of frustrations and failures as punctuation in an ongoing text. That is what gives you the opportunity to experience the elation of discovery, mastery, and conquest. Failure can become the starting-off point for a new beginning.

Do you try to get your needs met in all the wrong places? One lady I counseled was frustrated with her husband. She had unrealistic fantasies of being a princess, having her prince wine, dine, flirt, support, and caretake her forever after. It seems that she married a frog prince. He was critical, withdrawn, and demanding. We talked about her fears of growing up, being responsible, an autonomous individual who would share her life, rather than donate it to someone else's benevolent efforts. She complained, though, "What's so wrong about being dependent, about being a princess? Lots of women do that. They seem to make it work; why can't I?" That was an interesting question. You would think that if she truly wanted to be a princess, she would have married a bona fide prince type. She didn't. There's a reason why. Down deep, she didn't believe she was good enough to be treated well by anyone. Marrying a frog prince whom her friends and family disliked made her feel as though not being treated nicely had nothing to do with her. You often marry what seems like the wrong type that down deep solves a problem.

Do you always have the feeling you're missing something? Feeling like you're always missing something keeps you moving on to another territory, job, lover, philosophy, even style of clothes. As a therapist, I've seen so many people suddenly divorce, change careers, or find religion in the hopes of finally feeling fulfilled by having the ultimate. And then I've seen the devastating disappointment followed by yet another frenzied search. It is true that it often takes time to find your own way in life, a time filled with confusion and experimentation. Finding your own way, though, means you have to learn not only about yourself, but about life. Life offers choices. Choices are all like forks in the road. Something is discovered while something is left behind. Sometimes there are things missing from your life, yet sometimes what is missing is your own commitment and investment. So what you have becomes less meaningful and fulfilling regardless of its own characteristics. The next time you feel like something is missing, ask yourself if you've really explored what is there.

How can you survive anticipating the scary things you have to do? When you've got to make a speech, take a test, give a demonstration, or present a report, it makes you nervous. That's understandable. Being judged often impacts on your feelings of competency, value, and lovability. It's a hangover from childhood times when you were trying to impress your parents to get love and reassurance from them. How can you survive taking care of adult business with childhood apprehensions? Here are three choices: Instead of hinging everything about you on that one event, consider your existing worth to other people, which will not change because of this one experience. Second, you can focus in on the task itself—its meaning, its content, and your technique in handling it. In other words, take care of business. Third, you could remember or plan on something wonderful which will happen an hour or a day after this event, realizing that your life will go on, and quite well.

Whom must you be better than? One woman I counseled seemed to spend her whole life measuring her worth in looks, ability, and so on by comparing herself to others. Now, there are always others worse and better, but it was only the better ones that counted in her eyes. We tracked this need, these feelings, back into her childhood. She remembered that her brother was her mother's favorite. At least, it felt that way because her mother paid more attention and would always tell her to be just like her brother. In her child's mind, her mother favored the brother because she was not as good, as accomplished, as pretty. In other words, she took responsibility for her mother's behavior. Her mother may have been punishing her because the father was paying more attention to the little girl than to herself. Her mother's behavior probably had little to do with her personally. Yet the child's mind takes it personally and sometimes spends a lifetime trying to get Mother to finally love, accept, and approve.

Are you losing by intimidation? Are you hesitant to return something to the store? Do you hold back from complaining about poor food or service in a restaurant? Do you stew silently when someone cuts in line in front of you? Sometimes it's just not worth the effort and aggravation, and as long as you can let it go, perhaps even with humor, that's fine. If you're generally a pushover, sweatily frightened, or with an anger ulcer, it's time for you to ask yourself why everyone else's feelings are more important than yours. Why are your needs expendable? Why are you so invisible? It might be that you're still being a good little child of the barely seen and definitely not heard variety, or that you're still being a scared little child, afraid of everyone's frown of displeasure. People and situations often are unfair and selfish with or without intent. It's up to you to set the limits as to what you'll let pass and what you'll not. The end result is self-respect, a greater feeling of strength and value, and interestingly, more tolerance of others.

Do you plan life or play it by ear? Someone once said, "Life is what happens to you while you're making other plans." Some of you may feel that there is no point in planning your life because things seem to happen haphazardly and independently from your dreams and efforts. Some of you may feel that without plans, there is no hope for goals and dreams to be realized. You're both right. One of the myths of childhood is that good thoughts, good deeds, and persistence will get you the brass ring. Not necessarily, though some of you work compulsively trying to make it be so. One of the myths of adolescence is that if it's going to happen it will, so why bother worrying about it? Not necessarily, though some of you continue to sit out all the dances, still hoping to win the trophy. Disappointment might have made you cynical. Why try if there is no guarantee that life will give you what you want? What do you say to life when it gives you your plan and then you decide you want something else? Maybe there is something good about the flexibility.

What do you do with someone who's always giving you a hard time? You don't want to get into a tug-of-war with someone like that. People who are truly out to give you a hard time—out of envy, for instance—will be more committed to the war than you, and you will get decimated. First, distinguish between their giving you a hard time, undeserved, and their calling you to task for something you ought to take care of. If you're getting an unearned hard time, try ignoring it for a while. They might fizzle out with exhaustion or get distracted by someone or something else. If they don't, you've got to do something for your own protection. Their feelings of insecurity or inadequacy could lead them to treat you as a threat. Take the time, make the effort, to be a person with them. Perhaps that will relieve their anxieties and get them off your back. Try not to retaliate. Let significant others see you as a sincere, hardworking victim. You'll accumulate the appropriate allies.

Are you too easily intimidated? I was counseling a young woman who was working her way out of a lifetime of self-destructive behaviors—drugs, frequent impersonal sex, arrests, and physically brutal relationships. She generally felt weak and worthless, allowing people to use and abuse her, never being sure what was her right. Her early family experiences rarely supported her developing self-esteem or autonomy. The way she spent most of her life gave her little opportunity to develop these on her own. She finally had an experience she could tap into and use to support herself through difficult times. Her boss promised her a hundred dollars for a particular job. She did the job well. Without comment, he gave her ninety dollars. She didn't say anything. She went home angry. Maybe the job she did wasn't good enough. Maybe he'd get mad and fire her. Maybe she should leave her job. She decided to approach him calmly and matter-offactly and simply ask for the ten dollars more he owed her. He paid it immediately. She carries that ten-dollar bill with her all the time as a reminder of the strength and worth she's worked hard to give herself.

Why is it so hard for you to be a good loser? One man I was counseling was suffocating in the middle of his own paradox. He believed he had to win in order to be loved and approved of. Now, the paradox was that this meant he felt he had to one-up even his own loved ones to get their love. Needless to say, he mostly got their resentment. He was definitely a bad loser since losing meant more than just not being the victor. It meant reliving his childhood pain of disappointing his overly demanding parents. Losing, to him, threatened his sense of well-being and security as a child, even though he was now an adult. I don't think too many of you would really feel so bad about losing a game or an argument if on some level you wouldn't associate that with your value as a person or your lovableness and acceptability. When these are all connected, each game becomes a new time you test your being, rather than simply your skills, today. The broader-based your own sense of value is, the less likely that one or a few losses will be able to topple you.

Has life given you a raw deal? I do not doubt that life may have shortchanged you in some way—physical appearance, physical health, talents, breaks, nice family—but if you think for a moment that if any one of those things were different your whole life might be perfect, you might be right. It is in the thinking that things are okay, that they truly attain the status of okay. People who are happy don't generally get that way from enjoying the good luck they have benefited from. That's more a feeling of temporary relief. People who are happy over the long term become so because of that which they build themselves, even in the midst of adversity. Perfect moments are just that—moments. They're not to be sneezed at, but they're not to be counted on to add up to the sum total of your happiness. So you're right. Life has given you some bum raps. What are you going to do about it? Give up? Or consider this just the beginning of the game? Right now, consider something in your life you feel is unfortunate and unfair. Find a way to turn it into your advantage. I'll bet you can.

Are you often disappointed by the way people treat you? Maybe you're always going out of your way for people. You try always to anticipate people's feelings. You feel you're being exceptionally caring, yet time after time people hurt your feelings because they don't seem to be doing the same for you. You are expecting everyone in your life to go as far, do as much, as you are willing to. You also feel that you always do more and go farther than most people are willing to, and that's probably true. If you're feeling unworthy to receive, you might try to get recognition and satisfaction out of giving. When no one can match your magnanimity, you describe them as thoughtless. This way, you get yourself far away from that painful idea that you're not getting because you don't deserve to. It was all too easy for you as a child to distort and interpret many of your parents' behaviors as demonstrating a lack of love for you—if they were mad, sent you to camp, divorced, or died. Maybe it's time for you to settle those thoughts, fantasies, and feelings once and for all.

Where does confidence come from? I've heard people say, "I've got lots of confidence. I can do anything I set my mind to. If I want it, I'll get it." That's not confidence. That's a fantasy. It is not possible to do anything you want, no matter how hard you want it. You do have limits which involve the physical, mental, emotional, social, financial, and practical. If you're counting on cornering the market on success to ensure confidence, you're going to be sorely disappointed, and fast. I think confidence includes accepting the possibility of failure. Confidence has more to do with a willingness to face and survive adversity, embarrassment, and disappointment than with promising invincibility. You are more likely to allow yourself to try things if you don't put on yourself the awesome impossibility of always succeeding. In many cases you won't succeed, but the experience of the effort felt worth it.

Do you realize how much you're competing? Which would you more likely say: "I didn't do it as well as so-and-so" or "I didn't do it as well as I wanted to"? Do you forgive yourself by saying, "Oh, it's not much, but it's more than so-and-so has." Since there are always people better or worse off, you can always find a comparison with which to punish or satisfy yourself. What's behind that attitude? It may be habit. Remember always being compared to your brother or sister? "How come you aren't doing as well in school as John?" It may be an expression of your inner rage. When you best someone, do you feel elated, triumphant, vindicated, in some roundabout way? It may be that you have not evolved a sense of yourself as an independent being. You may feel as though you have no internal yardstick with which to measure or evaluate yourself. Your value is a function of whatever comparison is available. One thing's for sure, making comparisons doesn't ever make you happy, does it— compared to how happy you could be!

Do you need psychological "worming"? A tapeworm robs your body of the food it needs to stay healthy. A psychological tapeworm works the same way. No matter how much success or happiness you experience, it's not enough. There is a small tape in your head that says, "Uh-uh. You're still not good enough." So you struggle to do more, do better, never rest, never appreciate, never feel satisfied with yourself. You'll be better off without this tapeworm. You may think that without it you might not be motivated any longer. Wrong. That's the tapeworm talking, afraid to let you find out that accomplishing without end and without joy is empty and useless. Your psychological tapeworm tells you what you "should" do. Admit to yourself what you need and want. Here's where you get into trouble again, right? What you need and want is silly, selfish, childish. No. What you need and want is a part of what makes you unique, human, sensitive.

What's so bad about worry? Doesn't worry prove your depth of concern and sincerity? Doesn't worry show you are responsible in your concern about the future? Those are great rationalizations, but the answer to both questions is "no." When you worry constantly, you live in the land of "If." A land populated by failures, fears, hurts, betrayals, losses, shame, and even death. Successes and happy thoughts are rare accidents. There is power in worry. Those who love you don't want you to worry, so they give in to your fears and do whatever satisfies you. That gives you power to control them and them the need to maneuver around you. Learn to maneuver around yourself. Realize that worry is the way that you express your fears. Worry is your ticket away from risk and failure. Worry keeps you from being anything but a worrier. Worrying is not doing or being; it is suspended animation. How do you decide to quit worrying? Decide you're worth it.

Where and how did an ultimatum get such a bad reputation? Most respond to its issuance as though they were hit below the belt, as though it were dirty fighting or a nasty threat. An ultimatum is *supposed* to be a strong and final statement of intent and determination. It's supposed to make the point that idle bantering, bickering, and bellyaching are over. It's the time to make choices and moves. I think ultimata are more important to the ultimatum-er than the ultimatum-ee.

What usually keeps arguments and problems healthy
and alive is your fearful unwillingness to give credence
to your wants and live with the consequences of your
actions. So when you're finally willing to take a stand,
it could mean an effort toward increased self-respect
and esteem. Ultimata are therefore very serious.
Please don't waste them as vengeful weapons, nasties,
or idle threats. The focus of your self-image and your
life depends on it.

One of the reasons you're so stressed, looking so pale
and peaked and feeling so creaky, is that you're proud
of it. Notice how you're always talking about being
tired or achy or mind-blown, getting sympathy and
suggestions, but never persisting at changing anything. I worry that many of you are wearing tension
headaches, swigging antacid cocktails, and suffering
perpetual exhaustion because you're proud of what
you think it says. What does it say for you? That you
can challenge death and win? That you're so important and busy, you've got no time for mundane things
like rest and relaxation? That you take life seriously
and aren't selfishly frivolous? No. What it is really saying is that you're afraid—afraid that if you don't keep
going, going, going, you'll be gone off everyone else's
radar screen. It's mostly a measure of your anxieties

about self-worth, intimacy, loneliness, and death that keep you active past your own endurance, pleasure, and competency.

Does everyone say you're a pain in the neck? If everyone says you're a pain in the neck, maybe you are. Let's work from that assumption. Some of you pains in the neck behave so because you don't think you're going to be liked anyway, so why not be bratty, naggy, and pouty? The remedy might be to take some risks, carefully let down the barriers you have that keep others from knowing and liking you. Others of you are angry and hurt almost all of the time for reasons that escape even you. Everyone else, though, is made to pay for your pain. It might help for you to confront more directly your feelings of unattractiveness, intellectual drabness, or whatever notions of inadequacies haunt you. You pains in the neck are usually so because you feel hopeless and helpless to get recognized and reckoned with by any other means. It is time to risk. Learn new skills and change your image within yourself first. Others will catch the reflection. You pain-in-the-neck types could become tug-at-the-heart types.

Do you know how to say, "Thank you"? Are you one of those persons who upon getting a compliment wriggles your way out of it—"Well, I really wasn't so great," "Well, I really wanted it to come out differently," or some other such discounting of their gracious commendation? Don't think you're being so noble. First, you're being rude. Second, you're being self-punishing. Your inability to take a compliment may be a clear sign of your rotten self-image. You just can't seem to fathom that you could actually do something valid and valuable to another person. Some early training undermine your sense of your own value? Your immunity to compliments might also pinpoint a problem of perfectionism. That is, it isn't ever good enough, and it must be more than good enough before you are allowed to enjoy or take credit for it. Again, some early training? If you wear criticisms more comfortably than compliments, you're treating yourself like an errant child rather than a person who, like all of us, is just trying.

Are your feelings a kind of quicksand? You know what you should be doing, but you do what moves you at the moment anyway. Like when you're responding to the attention you're getting from a definite bad-news person: You realize the long-range potential dangers, but it feels so good to be noticed, to feel that someone likes you. You think you're willing to pay the price for that moment of joy, till your number is called. Then you're depressed and frustrated, wondering, "What's wrong with me?" What's wrong is that your immediate feelings are like quicksand. Whatever need or emotion you have at the moment is what you sink into like a security blanket. Your whole identity and self-esteem are built on these momentary pebbles rather than the firmer foundation of inner acceptance and inner faith which allows you to plan for the long run. The solution is to keep your sights on what you know to be right and good for you. Pull yourself out of those quicksand traps of immediate gratification of needs and take control of your life.

Do you find yourself checking out what you have or will say or do with others before you can feel settled? It's one thing to ask for advice or support on some issue; it's quite another to need all of that to even function. Just think of the pain you experience when you don't get it. My guess is that earlier in your life you made the decision to allow significant others in your family to feel more involved and important by giving them the gift of making up your mind for you, and now you're stuck in the habit. It's not that there's anything wrong in doing that; it's simply that your possibilities are limited. It would be nice, too, for you to be that strength for someone else and for yourself at times. To do that, you've got to believe your ideas and opinions are different from, but just as valuable as, everyone else's. No one really has cornered the market on wisdom.

So take their word for it! People telling you, "You're doing great," but you don't believe it? People telling you, "You're terrific," but you feel you know better? People telling you that they like you, but you don't feel likable? You resist all those compliments because you don't feel worthy and you worry, "What will happen when they really know the miserable, wretched truth about me?" This way of being must be driving you crazy! I've got an idea: Make believe they're right. Try living as though what they're saying is the truth. Maybe you are a bit likable and good at things. Could you dream of operating on the nice things people *do* say rather than your fantasies of the terrible things they *could* say? If you can, you might discover a new freedom and joy in life. Oh, I know what you're thinking. "It's all pretend. I'm really not that good and I know it." Maybe not. But 80 to 90 percent isn't bad, is it?

Feeling used is painful, unpleasant, and frustrating. It may also be your way. Allowing oneself to be used is an invitation to be misused—even if the other person isn't selfish or cruel. It's true only because your self-sacrifice is an exchange for getting something you aren't sure you deserve enough to ask for directly. And therein lies the true sadness and pain. If you asked for what you wanted and the other person said, "Don't be ridiculous, you worthless twit!" you would be living out your own worst nightmare. But if you give and give and give and give some more, and then obliquely request something, if it's turned down for any reason, then the other person is the twit and you are the victimized party. You forgive to try again. You forgive because the truth is, your low self-esteem says you weren't worth it anyway.

Do you get defensive too easily? When people offer you advice, suggestions, or even criticism, do you shoot before you see the whites of their eyes? That kind of reaction is defensive. It's an attempt to restore a sense of identity and value which you feel has been ripped away by their comments. How can a mere comment annihilate your identity or value? It can't.

Somehow, in your mind, the lack of complete approval and acceptance for each thing you do or say translates into a lack of approval and acceptance of you. When you were little, did you hear, "You did that, you bad boy!" or, "I can't love a child who does that"? Comments like these make children feel as though what they do is what they are. But doing something naughty or incorrect is not the same as being a bad person. Criticisms are never easy to swallow. We all want our show-and-tell to go well. But if you get all bent out of shape by criticism, you're taking the criticism too much to heart, like a dagger.

I know a lot of people who aren't as well off as a plastic ruler. You may be measuring yourself, your value, your very existence, by what you do. If you can take on ten challenges and get them all done, then you feel good about yourself. If you turn a project down or don't get it done right or on time, your value diminishes. If this sounds like you, then you're a person who never says "no" to the requests of others, and you'll always put work first. Now think of one of those plastic rulers you had when you were a kid in school. The first thing you notice is that it is a bit over a foot long. Imagine placing it against something you'd like to measure. Aha! Six inches long. Look again at the ruler. Even though it is working on measuring something six inches long, it stays its original length of twelve inches. The identity of the ruler has stayed the same regardless of its task. Yours is dependent upon your task, as though you were still performing for your parents' approval. You've made their approval the day-by-day, minute-by-minute calculation of your worth and identity. Try being a ruler.

Ever notice how you take too much garbage from people? Maybe it takes a bit of wheedling or manipulating, but most people know that if they work on you in just the right way, you'll give in. No matter what they've done or how often they've done it to you, you seem to have a perpetual capacity to take it. On the one hand, it seems so noble of you to be so incredibly tolerant of others' misbehaviors. On the other hand, you're starting to look like a glutton for punishment. What is this about? At least two things. First, you may get angry, and quite justifiably, you think. Then the doubts begin. "Maybe it's my fault. Maybe this really isn't so bad as I think." So you take away the justification for your anger. Second, you suffer over the potential loss of people more than you do over the constant affront to you. Somewhere, you've lost the sense of yourself as competent, valuable, and worth better treatment. If so, it's time to find yourself. Rebuild your self.

# CHAPTER 6

# Emotional Honesty

Are you anguished when you should be angered? When people are being a pain in the neck, do you try to please and placate? What comes next? Do you take out your frustrations on yourself or uninvolved others? Or do you just keep it all inside? Let me guess what comes next. Headaches, stomachaches, intestinal frenzies, and heart palpitations, right? No good. You've got to change your responsive anguish, which is killing you, into anger—appropriately expressed anger in the form of direct, honest assertiveness. Screaming at loved ones because others are driving you crazy does not solve the problem or get rid of the tension. Screaming at those problem people might create more problems. Realize first that you aren't facing your difficulties head-on, probably because you're afraid of seeming mean, rotten, or unlovable. Direct, honest, and assertive is not mean, rotten, or unlovable. The quality of your life depends on your accepting that.

How do you cope with unreturned favors? How many times have you done nice things for people and not gotten a "thank you," much less a returned favor? If it's happened too often with the same people, then you'd better check your choice of friends, as well as your motivation to be giving in such a selfish atmosphere. You're trying to make the wrong people like you by sacrificing more and getting less. However, the experience of giving and never receiving even politeness is universal. Some of you turn sour on the whole thing, deciding never to go out of your way again. Others keep trying, hoping that the other person will eventually discover some manners or thoughtfulness. Still others of you attempt to escape the dilemma by trying to believe that it is only the giving that counts. Friendship is an exchange, an interaction. Exchanging secrets and platitudes is not enough to sustain and nurture friendship. Frankness is important. Ever so gently, tell your friend you're disappointed, that you would have liked whatever it is. Don't hide, withdraw, or attack. Express yourself.

Do you feel guilty doing nothing? Is it really possible to do nothing? Ever try to remember something or figure something out and find yourself up against a brick wall? It was when you stopped pounding on it, when you just let your body and mind go limp, that an insight, an idea, a memory came to you. It's an exciting feeling, and it happens when you are ostensibly doing nothing. Some of the greatest discoveries and creative experiences have come to people when their mind was the most receptive, at apparent rest. There is an image, however, that to do something you have to be feverishly active. What you really need is for your mind to be receptive, and that requires you to be unstressed. This argument about rest still focuses on accomplishment and activity, albeit subtle activity. What is so wrong with "bumming off," doing nothing? From whence comes the guilt for simply experiencing your breathing or the sound of dust settling on the table? Why are these efforts without intrinsic value? Why do you need to have some concrete justification for them? You answer that.

Do you always have to see it to believe it? I'm not saying you've got to be some kind of gullible, naive, totally dependent wimp, but really, does everything people tell you have to be confirmed or refuted firsthand? Obviously, if something affects you, it's important to be careful. Where is your dividing line between responsible awareness and a frightening lack of trust? If you really think your beloved is almost totally unreliable, I question your motivation in choosing such a partner. If, instead, you can't ever feel comfortable trusting another with anything having to do with your welfare, emotional or physical, then it would seem that your childhood experiences led you to the conclusion that life's structure and security must come from you. While it may make you feel powerful, superior, and dominant to have your finger on everything going on, it does little to make others appreciate you, and it does little to make you feel secure enough to give your heart over to the tender ministrations of those who love you.

What is winning? In the film version of *Robinson Crusoe* with Peter O'Toole, there was a terrific lesson about winning. He was teaching Friday about civilization. This day's lesson was on competition and winning. He set up a running course and explained to Friday that they had to run from the beginning to the end as fast as they could. The first one to the end was the winner. The race began. Robinson Crusoe was shown straining, pumping, sweating, grimacing, in pain, pushing as hard as he could, and Friday was hopping, skipping, giggling, twisting in the air, having a good ol' time. Crusoe got to the finish line first, proclaiming his win, and chastising Friday for not doing it right. Friday disagreed, saying, "I won the race. I won because I had a good time doing it. Your face is all

crunched up, in pain. Is that what you call winning?"
How many things are there in your life you don't enjoy
because you have to win, win more than anything?
Maybe you've been losing more than you realized.

I'd like you to try my good part, bad part game. My
good part, bad part game is very easy. Take anything
good and say the bad parts. Take anything bad and say
the good parts. Here are some examples. Something
good: You got a big break at work. The good parts are
obvious. The bad parts may be that now you have
more responsibility, less free time, more problems to
solve, greater visibility for criticism, and maybe less
security. I know that sounds like a downer thing to do
to the good news, but hang in. Now, something bad:
You've lost something valuable. The bad part's obvious. The good parts: Well, you finally realized how
much it meant to you to find yourself reminiscing
warmly over it. You plan to be more vigilant and careful with valuables. You think about how important
you've made things rather than experiences and people, and so on. The punch line is that good and bad
things have much in common. They are both two-
sided and contain each other. Putting them both in
perspective with my good part, bad part game may
help you survive painful unhappinesses and ward off
painful disappointments.

Why is it you go after what you say you don't want? One man I was counseling was adamant. "I want a lady in my life who is warm, open, affectionate, and very huggy," he said. He described the women in his life as cold, withdrawn, and demanding. When I brought his current wife into the counseling, I noticed something interesting. Whenever she would express warmth or tenderness, he would shut it off, sometimes by starting another fight, ignoring or refuting the sincerity of her behavior. It seemed as though he were avoiding the very warmth and lovies he spoke about wanting. His original family had been a hardworking crew who never acknowledged overt, tender feelings. His longing for those experiences, together with his lack of comfortable familiarity with them, resulted in his shying away from them. You may say you're dying for intimacy or affection, yet find yourself behaving contrariwise. That's generally because your heart yearns and your fear churns, fear usually winning out. Rather than blaming others, work on making the unknown more familiar.

If you could be reincarnated into a thing, what thing would you choose to be and why? One man said, "A

teddy bear so that people could hug me. Most people
expect me to take care of them." Interesting. Most of
the time, he looks like a confident papa bear. People
have learned what to expect from him because he's
trained them. One woman said, "A boulder, so that
things would either smash into me and break up or
splash and bounce by me. Either way, I wouldn't get
hurt by things and people so much anymore."
Interesting. Most of the time, she looks like a sponge,
absorbing pain and problems in a martyrish way. One
young boy said, "A football, so that people could play
with me and have fun." Interesting. Here was a lonely
little boy whose parents were using him for an emotional football in their brutal divorce skirmishes. He,
somehow, felt responsible, helpless, powerless, and in
the middle. If you could be reincarnated into a thing,
what thing would you choose to be and why? Answer
this question, and I promise you'll learn a lot about
feelings you've been tucking away.

Is your body paying the price for your emotional
pain? Is it stomachaches, headaches, exhaustion,
heart palpitations, sweaty palms, intestinal frenzies?
What part of your body expresses your emotional
pain? Think of it as a trade-off. It's both a conscious
and an unconscious bargain you've made with yourself. You're not wanting to risk and feel some particular experience, like the vulnerability of directness, so

you hold back. If that would resolve the situation for you, that would be fine. If that would resolve your conflicted feelings, that would be fine. When it does neither, the pain often becomes translated into a physical symptom. That physical symptom might not be a totally negative experience for you. Perhaps it gets you a special kind of attention, support, and permissiveness. Even if you feel ashamed of that, it's real and it's hard to give up. That physical symptom, though, is also a reminder that there is something in your life you're not handling in your own best interest.

Do you hate game playing? Many of you despise game playing. You say you hate having to "kiss up," to be friendly when you don't feel like it, to give compliments you don't believe in, to spend time chatting that you know could be spent better. You feel the charade shouldn't be necessary. People should do things for you because you're splendid, correct, sincere, and good. Perhaps what you call playing games is not selling your soul, after all. Perhaps it's simply being courteous, friendly, gracious, and classy. Sometimes working very hard at becoming makes you forget or discount the importance of being. Becoming marvelous at something does not make you the center of everyone's universe. It does give you the opportunity to give special things to people. If you want to be sup-

ported in giving your specialness, you've got to recip-
rocate, often in advance, by being sensitive to the subtle specialness of others. If this is game playing,
remember how much fun and mutually satisfying a
pleasant game can be.

Do you hold on to the past? As a therapist, I'm aware
of what people are telling me when they come in for
their first session, complaining bitterly about previous
therapists. In part, they may be telling me of some inappropriate and hurtful behaviors of those therapists.
In part, they are telling me of their personal sensitivities and, in part, they are warning me about what they
will and will not tolerate from me. Do you find yourself
constantly reiterating old hurts and treachery of your
family, prior lovers, friends? Is it truly that you simply
can't forget, or haven't gotten all the pain out yet?
Might it be that remembering old pain serves a new
purpose? Your old pain might be the way you manipulate your present partners or friends into being especially solicitous, tolerant, or careful. It also might be
the way you get yourself off the hook for not being
more giving, less selfish. If you're doing this and it's
working, it won't last. Lasting love will come your way,
not in exchange for your past hurts, but in exchange
for present lovingness.

Is it so bad to take the easy way out? When you think of the easy way out, what comes to mind? Being chicken? Copping out? Running away? These are mostly negative in sentiment, implying weakness and the lack of intestinal fortitude. Definite no-no's. Assertiveness, confrontiveness, and directness are admired. But all of those notions only take *you* into account. How about the other party? What if it were more in his emotional or situational interest for you to take the so-called easy way out? Would it still be a sign of weakness on your part? If so, would that be the only or most important issue? You may be too concerned with how you look or how you would seem and not concerned enough about the totality of the circumstance for everyone involved. It might be more humane to work around the confrontation or morbid complexity involved in handling this situation more directly. Perhaps there are other ways of backing off. The easy way out might be so for everyone.

Do you long to be free? Do you fantasize about not having any more work or responsibilities? Having your partner evaporate? Having your family off your back? This reminds me of a *Twilight Zone* episode. A man hated people, didn't want to be bothered by anyone or anything. He got his wish, and shifted into a state of existence without connection to the world. His loneliness overwhelmed him. No doubt that kids and spouses can be pains. No doubt that work can sometimes overwhelm. No doubt that everything can look grim. Fantasizing about total freedom from all of it may seem like the best solution. Think again. There are some things you would miss—aspects of challenge, reward, emotional return. Fantasizing about total freedom is a total annihilation of so much you've built and sacrificed for. When you fantasize, you stay in the same place, building up more and more resentment. There are alternatives—changes in scheduling or the ways you operate, changes in attitude, changes in balancing between fun and work. Escape to total freedom requires great losses. Changes bring you greater freedom without losses.

Do you often leave without going? One young man I was counseling was worrying about his attacks of crazies. He said he'd be with people in some particular circumstance and find himself in some other space, not himself. That this happened would upset and anger him. He was worried about being crazy. I was worried that he might believe that. Among other things, life is an ongoing sequence of trade-offs. If you're tall, you can't be short, and if you're being crazy at the moment, you can't be facing what feelings and thoughts are frightening you. So perhaps having an attack of the crazies is a kind of protection. When this young man and I explored the circumstances that precipitated his crazies, we discovered that they would happen whenever he felt emotionally vulnerable. Instead of working through the situation at the moment, his mind would switch into crazy gear, although his feet kept him in the situation where he role-played to please the other person. The key to reducing his attack of the crazies was to have him face the truth—the truth of his feelings at the moment and the truth of the person he was with.

Do you know why you take out your frustrations on the ones you love? If you take out your frustrations on the ones you hate, you won't get the same attempt at tolerance and understanding you get from your loved ones. If you take out your frustrations on people you don't know, it could be dangerous. If you take out your frustrations on yourself, it hurts too much. Actually, there is even more involved. When you complain, rant, rave, stomp, pound, accuse, attack, and demand, you may really be asking for something. That something could be a magical fix-it-up. It could be a coded cry for reassurance that both you and life are not really that hopeless. If your loved ones are getting fed up taking the flak for your frustrations and you're starting to feel more and more like an impulsive maniac, there is a way to change. Whatever has happened has caused you to feel a certain way, maybe hurt, frightened, dumped, or dumped on. Whatever it is, identify it and say it out loud. "I feel dumped and I'm hurt and angry." Now your loved ones have something to offer.

Complain, complain, complain! What for? Good grief! You complain a lot about her, him, the situation. The way you go on, I can't imagine anyone putting up with all you do. And yet, when I look closer, you're not making sure anything changes or trying to get out of the situation. Very interesting. One woman I was counseling complained that her husband beat her. He wouldn't come in for therapy. She wouldn't get out of the relationship. It turned out that she thought herself lucky, in a sad way, that he didn't beat her nearly as much as her father had. She was counting this as a blessing. A young man in therapy complained furiously about how his girlfriend ran hot and cold, confusing and frustrating him. He would complain, fume, and cry during the bad times. When she ran hot again, he was in seventh heaven. He was grateful to have someone want him even periodically. You complain, not without justification, yet you don't follow it up with action, such as demands for redress or an announcement of an ultimatum, because you don't see yourself as deserving or getting more.

Do you think having or showing emotions is bad? You can probably think of too many times you were made to feel weak, bad, or the loser just because you got emotional. You might remember being taught not to let the other person know they had gotten to you because they'd gloat. Maybe you've been told it isn't mature, masculine, or professional to show emotions. I watch the TV news a lot. On one channel, I saw an anchor going from a story about a murder to a tease about a local music trend, all with the same half smile. On another news program, I saw how deeply touched the anchor was after a news story about a child losing a valiant fight against leukemia. That's the station I continue to watch. If someone feels triumphant because they were able to get you to show emotional pain and upset, why not give them their victory? After all, what have they won? A debate about which one of you feels deeply? Which one of you dares to risk open vulnerability? Visible emotion doesn't automatically mean you've lost your intelligence, your will, competency, responsibility, or direction. It means you're a sensitive human being.

Feeling it isn't the same as doing it. One young man I know had been beaten by his father throughout his entire childhood. His mother never protected him or herself from his father's drunken rages. And now, as an adult, he is afraid of relationships, openness, and even happiness. He lives in fear of what he sees as the two parts of himself: his weakness, which could make him vulnerable to being victimized again, and his strength, which he worries might make him overdo it just like his dad. What does this extreme situation have to do with you? Have you had a thought, a feeling, an urge that shocked or scared you? Maybe scared you so much you were afraid to feel, think, or act or even tell anyone about it? It might have had to do with sex, need, love, hate, fear, or revenge. The young man I mentioned listened to his own voices of avenger and victim and realized that those were only two of many creative and loving voices. Thinking it, feeling it, doesn't mean he didn't have control over what to be.

What, me worry? You say, "It's not going to happen to me." Then it does. Then come the regrets of not having been more careful, not having planned. Sometimes there is another chance, sometimes not. There is something to positive thinking. That attitude may help you avoid disasters—sometimes. Other times, this positive thinking of yours may be camouflage for your fears of facing reality. You may not want to think of death, yet you don't use your seatbelt. You may not want to think of pregnancy, yet you don't use a contraceptive. On the other hand, you could worry and plan yourself right out of any positive experiences, successes, and enjoyment. And you could underworry and plan yourself right out of any positive experiences, successes, and enjoyment. Not facing your fears doesn't keep them from happening. It just keeps you from participating in your own life.

Feel embarrassed to mourn the death of your pet? Somebody tell you that you're silly for getting overemotional about your pet dying? They tell you that, after all, it's only an animal; you can always get another one. Do you apologize for still having sobbing sessions whenever you remember your bird taking seed from your pocket, your cat lying on your chest when you were in bed with a cold, your dog snuggling close when you were feeling low? You don't need to apologize or feel silly about missing an animal that accepted you without question, an animal whose attention, loyalty, and love reminded you of the more gentle, peaceful, human side of yourself. You and your pet had a special relationship. Those frustrations, irritations, and inconveniences which are a part of taking care of an animal now seem to transform into anecdotes which make you chuckle and choke up. The depth of your pain measures the depth of the love you had, love still available to be given to yet another eager sweet animal.

I was counseling a sixty-two-year-old woman whose forty-year marriage was coming to an end. For her, it was as though her life were coming to an end, and she fought. Her weapons? Tears, suicide threats, demandingness, the punishing of all those who tried to help her. Why? Because when you accept their help, you are accepting the reality of why you need their help. All of it. The tears, the threats, the misbehaviors are all desperate attempts to push back reality, deny change, hurt back for your hurts. Those close to you need to understand so that they can get through what might be a necessary, terrible period of denial, hurt, and anger. You need to understand so that you can know that your feeling this way won't last.

Aging getting to you? Notice that your body is creaking and pooching out in places it didn't use to, no matter what you do to prevent it? Notice people respond to you differently? Have different expectations of you? It's easy to be disappointed in yourself because you thought at this age you'd have or be doing what you're not. These are normal feelings, and they are real issues to resolve. Maturing isn't just getting wiser with the situation you have at the moment. It's learning how to adapt to situations changing over time and mostly not within your control. Aging is sometimes cruel, and its challenge is to health and functioning. But your most dangerous enemy is seeing aging as an enemy. That will put you in constant pain, sorrow, and war. When would you then enjoy where and who you are? When would you experience those things worth celebrating, worth remembering? Aging is not an enemy. It's only life.

Someone wrote and asked me if I thought it was normal to believe that you could be happy only if you had such great success that you could go back to your high school reunion and say, "Eat your hearts out, suckers." This reminded me of someone I was counseling who said, "What does it mean that I get more satisfaction out of the failures of others than the successes of myself?" Wanting others to be jealous as a source of your happiness is really the flip side of the same sentiment. It's all about envy. And envy is a mean emotion. It means you feel lessened by other people's accom-

plishments and imagine that they respond in kind.
People who envy wish the worst for others and are relieved only when that wish comes true. Envy comes
out of your own feelings of deprivation, loneliness, and
emotional need. Happiness is never yours. Yours is the
relief when others are not happy either. So, to answer
your question, whether you're normal isn't even the
point. That you'll never find happiness through others' lack of it is the point.

"Then what?" Do you find yourself not saying something or doing something because you're afraid of the
outcome? It probably only helps you feel even more
alone and frustrated, right? There's an old saying
about the devil you know and the devil you don't
know. The devil you know is supposed to be the easier
one to deal with; at least you know what to expect. It
just might be that you can face some of your fears the
same way. Imagine you want to tell someone something and you're afraid. Start asking the question,
"Then what?" In doing this, you will move from the
devil you don't know to the one you do. Let's try it. If I
take a class, I might not do well. Then what? I'll get a
bad grade. Then what? Uhm. It always gets harder as
you go along. Well, people in class will know. Then
what? At this point, you may run out of answers and
discover that the devil you know doesn't really seem
very important at all.

Don't bother with the small stuff. People have probably told you your whole life, "That's not important enough to be upset about." If that gets you angry, there are two possibilities: they are right or they're wrong. If they're right, then you are really angry with yourself for having no priority system that selects out those issues or situations really worthy of your grief and aggravation. If they're wrong, then you're dealing with people to whom you have not adequately communicated your feelings. Or they think their feelings should be everybody's. As in most of life, there are lots of possibilities. And it is for that reason that you must allow yourself the luxury of standing back and picking and choosing more carefully that which you are willing to come all unglued about. Not only that, getting unglued may not be the only alternative. Sometimes letting things just pass might be good. Sometimes a gentle confrontation, sometimes a long-range plan, makes being upset only a part of your emotional repertoire.

"I can't believe I feel that way. What kind of person am I?" One woman I counsel said that her newborn, severely handicapped child had died. She was in such terrible pain, she couldn't sleep because of the night-mares. Mourning the death of a child is very special pain. You feel responsible and guilty for not being able to protect someone so dependent and vulnerable. This young woman felt intense loss for her child, and she felt like a failure for not being able to give birth to a healthy child. And she secretly also felt some relief at not having to face a life with a handicapped child. Horrified that she could even think such a thing, she psychologically defended against what she felt was an unacceptable, negative feeling by experiencing in-tense, intractable pain. It's natural. It's human to have both negative and positive feelings about anyone or anything, especially something intimate and sensitive. Sometimes you need to be reminded to accept your humanness.

Ever feel like you just don't want to do something? Everyone tries to do heavy analysis on the deep signif-icance of your lack of interest. It's interesting, maybe even correct. Nonetheless, you just don't want to do it. Shouldn't that be respected? I think so. The trap is one of defending and explaining. You're always going to get caught up in those confusions. Then you get angry. Then there are fights. Then you can't even enjoy not doing whatever it is you don't want to do. I think the main problem is that you don't respect the simpler motivations you have. You're thinking that to justify your inaction, it's got to be some big, heavy deal. Hey, don't put that pressure on yourself. If the truth is that you are just too tired, too spent, say it. If the truth is that you're afraid, say it. If the truth is that it simply doesn't matter enough to you to justify the effort, say it. You now have two things available: you understand yourself better and you can enjoy not doing whatever it is because it's out in the open.

How should you handle a person who is jealous or envious of you ? What's your first gut reaction to someone else's not-too-veiled envious behavior toward you? There are several commen reactions. One is panic that you aren't going to be liked anymore. Or worse, that you are going to be harmed in some way. Those reactions generally come from some guilt feelings about having more than someone else and perhaps feeling responsible for their unhappiness. Maybe your reaction is to gloat. That reaction comes out of your enviousness. Joy that someone else has less comes from the same place as sadness that someone else has more. Someone else's envy is his unfortunate problem; don't let it be yours to be happy by or responsible for. Don't placate, don't feed it.

Is compromise really a good idea? When one of you wants it one way and the other wants it a different way, compromising somewhere in the middle is supposed to bring you happily together. Does it? Nope. Not if compromising means you have to give up or take up something against your true wishes and feelings. It may not show immediately, or even directly, but your resentment will eventually seep through. Sometimes you fake it. You pretend to agree to a compromise solution to appear to be the reasonable one, or so that you can escape the conflict. Unfortunately, your resentments continue to percolate. Giving up or giving in, by themselves, do not bring people closer together. You and your partner would feel more okay about giving up something if you both felt there was something even more important to gain—like good feelings between you or respect for one another's emotional needs. Without those as part of the bargain, the deal will never be satisfying.

Do you get the kind of response you'd really like from your dearly beloved? One woman complained about her husband's lack of response when she was explaining to him her ideas about working through a problem with their son. "He listened and nodded and said, 'I think you're right,'" she explained. "I was so angry." She realized that she wanted something more or different from him. She wasn't sure what. But her being angry with him was really her frustration with herself aimed outward. When you don't want to admit something to yourself, it is difficult to expect the other to respond to that something with anything useful. This woman was feeling insecure about her ideas and needed affirmation of their rightness. However, when she spoke it was with the authority of a confident person. She did that to mask her fears and vulnerability. You need to express that scary truth before you can expect to get any help with it.

# CHAPTER 7

# *Self-realization*

Are you a human eraser? There are those who go through life trying to leave their mark, and there are those who go through life trying to erase the marks of others. Which are you? By "leaving your mark," I'm not talking about graffiti; I mean taking risks, being creative, adventurous, useful, meaningful, standing out and standing up. That means being vulnerable to criticism, attack, frustration, and failure. Beware of being a human eraser. That's someone who can't stand to see someone accomplish, shine, or excel. That someone is you if you gain relief from undermining or demeaning someone else's mark on life. Since you are afraid to make your own mark, you erase the marks of others. You eliminate that telltale contrast which you worry would highlight your laziness or unworthiness or whatever else you feel you are. The next time you criticize or put down someone else's efforts, ask yourself whether or not you secretly wish you were that person. If you do, then help him or her and explore your fears of being a human marker, rather than a human eraser.

How do you deal with your envy? When you envy, you begrudge the well-being and success of others. It's hard to admit to, but you do it. Your envy shows when you search for faults among the laurels of their triumph. Your envy shows when you struggle for some way to diminish their success. That means that you see life as having a finite amount of anything, so if someone has more, someone else automatically has less. As for envy, your emotional reaction to another's success is that you see yourself as less. In diminishing them, you rise again in value. This state of mind makes you a human barometer of self-worth, rising and falling with what is going on around you. As long as no one else's head rises above the crowd, you have safety from negative feelings about yourself, even if you're steeped in mediocrity. Life doesn't have to be a perpetual competition. It can be an opportunity for your personal satisfaction.

Do you drive through life looking only through the rearview mirror? I'll bet there have been too many times you've wanted to start something new or change direction, but didn't. Even the thought of it made you feel guilty. There are lots of philosophical tidbits we nibbled as kids which contribute to these guilts. Don't start anything you're not going to finish, or don't start something new till you're finished, and stick with whatever you start. When you're growing up and learning discipline, these are helpful. When you don't feel comfortable with flexibility, then these helpful words have become tyrannical. One thing all those sayings leave out is the benefit of experience. Starting something new, learning it, and then going on to something else does not necessarily mean that what you've done is lost or meaningless. It means you've learned things which have allowed you to expand your horizons and abilities. It's additive, not subtractive. Allow yourself to grow to new challenges, relishing and using the experience of past ones.

Do you have ugly days? You know what ugly days feel like. No matter what anybody says about how you look or how you're handling things, you just feel ugly and yucky anyway. You can't be reasoned, humored, or browbeaten out of this mood. It has to run its course. What is this feeling ugly business about? It has to do with frustration and depression. When you are up past your eyeballs with things not going the way you want and you don't have any sense of control or hope, all of that gets turned toward the only person you're able to get to, you. Ugly days are the way you cope with outer frustrations by literally becoming the ugliness you can't overcome. Looking in the mirror and saying "yuck" and looking at your work and saying "yuck" are examples of displaced anger, hurt, and helplessness. Having ugly days now and then is not a particular problem. Having more ugly days than not is a sign of your emotional frustration turning into self-destruction.

Do you discard friends? Are you amazed when someone tells you that they've had this friend for at least half or a whole lifetime? Are you suspicious when someone seems to be working hard at making or maintaining a friendship with you? Do you sometimes feel incredibly alone when you need help and there's no one to call? Perhaps that loneliness will motivate you to look inside yourself and understand your prejudice and flippancy about friends and friendship. Not having friends or disposing of friends is your way of avoiding something. To discover what that something might be, let's look back in your life. Did your parents enjoy friendship so that you had positive role models of sharing, caring, and trusting, or did they warn you not to say too much to people lest it be used against you? Did you and your siblings have friendships growing up, or were competition, put-downs, setups, and betrayals the whole menu? Did you feel like you fit in with your school chums? Your early experiences with friendships have a profound impact on you now—how much you'll risk, how much you'll trust, and how much you'll be alone.

What do you admire about yourself the most? You're supposed to be displaying great humility, honesty, and courage when you're willing to list your faults and foibles. It's not so bad talking about bad tempers and insecurity when you're getting supported and stroked for it. It's not easy to get the same support and stroking for talking about your magnificence. There's a lot of guilt surrounding tooting your own horn. That lack of humility is considered by some to be unpardonably sinful. I feel it's only considered bad by insecure people who need to feel that you're no better than they. Those people need others homogenized into mediocrity to maintain any sense of personal well-being. There is nothing wrong with your appreciating what you have, what you've done, and who you are. It's the kind of loving awareness that you can share and give to others. Start now. Do you admire your guts, your accomplishments, your sensitivity? You've earned it.

Is even play work for you? Do you jog and play tennis
or cards with the same ferocity that you bring to
work? Do you have the same desperate drives toward
rigor, discipline, and perfection? Does your approach
to play leave you tickled and relaxed or exhausted and
frenzied? When I say the word "play," you probably
picture a child doing what children are supposed to
do. When you think of yourself at play, you may think
it's silly, childish, a waste of time, nonproductive, lazy,
and a definite no-no for someone of your caliber. You
are living under a tyranny that dictates that you
should always be productive and perfect at it. You,
most likely, accept relaxation only in the context of
reward for all tasks completed or acceptable only in
illness. What made the notions of feeling good and
having fun or fooling around at something so disdain-
ful, so unjustifiable as a natural, normal, reasonable,
valuable part of being alive? A lot depends upon your
working that out: your family relationships, friendships, health, the quality of your own existence.

What makes it hard for you to accept help? Notice
how good you are about giving advice and assistance
to others, yet whether you complain about it or not,

*you* seem to weather things alone. That's not accidental. It's your design. Somewhere along the line, you
learned that needing help meant taking abuse, being
overwhelmed, controlled, used, ignored. Whatever the
case, you've become incredibly self-protective, relying
on yourself. Maybe you take care of others partially to
hint to them about what you'd like. Nonetheless, it's
still hard for you to trust receiving the help. Don't
trust unless you're sure of the following two factors:
First, do you think the person is reasonably trustworthy? That means, will he try to do the best by you?
Look at him clearly, not through the lenses of past disasters. Second, do you think you can survive the disappointment should he inadvertently mess things up?
Think about this. Don't let the hurts of the past keep
you from being loved now.

Do you work harder for failure than success? Do you
get to a point of potential success and comfort, and
then *poof,* something happens and it's all gone? You
start climbing again, only to have the same thing happen. One couple's business would start to take off, and
before they knew it, their spending was ahead of their
earning. Their management skills seemed to evaporate, and the business collapsed again and again. We
talked about budgeting accountants and better man-
agers, all the obvious things. It seemed to me, though,
that there was a deeper meaning to the repetitive fail-

ure. Indeed there was: guilt. When they were first
starting out together and things were tough, they had
done some illegal and emotionally wrenching things to
survive. The deep guilt they felt kept them from accepting success. Unconsciously, they both felt they
deserved to be punished for what they did. Consciously, they felt what they did was necessary. The
unconscious won, and they doomed themselves to a
life of punitive failures. What are you punishing yourself for with your failures?

Are you afraid you're crazy? Many of you have parents
who seem deeply emotionally disturbed. It's not un-
common for offspring to worry if they, too, will have
emotional problems. If you've been worrying about
that and not facing it openly, you may be doing some
destructive things to yourself and your loved ones.
One woman hated her mother, mostly because she
feared her mother's mental illness. Without admitting
it to herself, she worried that she might become just
like her mom. She got married and had a little girl. In
subtle ways, she tormented that child, being too critical, only meaning to be instructive; withholding love
and affection, only meaning to avoid spoiling her. The
little girl's behavior began to look crazy. In a way, the
mother was relieved, unconsciously feeling safe because the craziness she feared was not in herself; it

was in her daughter. If you have that fear, you might not allow yourself a steady job or relationship, lest your imagined craziness become manifest and you be rejected. Your fears are not necessarily reality. Face them.

Let's not forget about luck. If you're one to get down on yourself when things don't go right, you may not be entirely fair. The right time, place, and situation are as important to success as ability. Now, don't take that as a further indictment of yourself. You don't have control over time, place, and situation. Don't forget that your life is intersecting with the lives of others. Each of you has goals, dreams, needs, abilities, and special interests. It may be difficult for you to see that the world and the people in it don't particularly operate for the benefit or deficit of your interests. The world just is. It may be that you attain your one special dream. It may be that you don't. Is the entirety of your life going to be sacrificed for that one end? Is that the totality of your worth? Is that really the only way you can be happy? If your answers to all of those are "no," then you've got a great chance for a good life. If your answers to some of those were "yes," then you've got little chance for inner peace and satisfaction.

Do you feel all washed up? You've been focused on a dream, and it's all become a disappointing blur. At this point, it's easy to feel like your life has no meaning or that it's over. This despair is like a dark, thick filter. No rays of positiveness, no appreciation of the good things your efforts have developed, get through. If this is where you are now, I'm not going to be able to rationalize you out of it. I'll bet those who know and love you have tried. You may have met their efforts with pained anger, telling them they don't understand, and you're right; it is difficult to understand this level of desperate hopelessness unless you're immersed in it or remember your own last bout with it. I imagine you're going to stay with these feelings for a while, praying for a miracle or a benevolent fairy godmother, someone to rescue you or fight your battle. Then you're going to go on with some new attitudes and insights about your life. If you'll let it happen, you're going to be okay.

You've tried it. What makes changing so difficult? When you finally get down on your humbles, you realize that there are some changes you could stand to make. Now that you're not being defensive, you even notice you could benefit from those changes. Since it's all so straightforward, simple, and clear, why do you have such a hard time even starting, much less sustaining those changes? Obvious, simple, beneficial, are not enough. The final ingredient is an understanding of how important it's been for you all these years not to change. Generally, styles of behavior that could stand renovation are defensive behaviors. Those are ways you had to learn to survive some difficult times in your life, perhaps during childhood. These were the times when flexibility, testing, and stretching yourself were too dangerous. By now, those defenses are habit. The part of changing that is often overlooked is the learning and adapting required to change defending into facing and coping. Only then will changing that habit come more naturally.

Are you too easily intimidated? Some people work at being intimidating. Some are intimidating by circumstance. Uniforms, power, physical size, loudness, and arrogance all are factors for potential intimidation. A healthy respect for factors of power or position is realistic and practical. A perpetual feeling of intimidation is not. Your feelings of intimidation suggest that you see yourself within everyone's power, that they can make you do or feel their will, that you are dependent upon them for your very personhood. Sexual harassment, for example, has these elements. You feel that if you don't respond positively to your superior's advances, you'll lose your job. If you lose your job, you can sue. If you lose yourself, then momentary security has more importance than your own integrity and emotional well-being. Momentary security becomes that vital when you feel generally powerless, incompetent, and unworthy to take care of yourself. You are again as a child, dependent upon yet another parent.

Perhaps your greatest weakness is your fear of being weak. Do you refuse to cry in front of anyone, lest someone think you weak? Do you refuse to ask for help, lest someone see you as weak? Do you hold in your pain, lest someone know you're weak? So you withdraw to hide and intimidate to push away, all the time convincing yourself that you're right because your way is superior, and still you're frightened and unhappy. Weakness, as a blessing or a sin, probably isn't the real issue with you. It isn't a moment of weakness you fear. It is the sense that you have no strength to tap into, really, so that if you let down, even for a moment, you might regress finally and for all time into the blob of defenseless helplessness you imagine yourself to be. Children are all defenseless and helpless. Were you used and abused or supported and nurtured during those weak years? Those experiences taught you about trusting others with power or advantage

over you, and also about the comfort of being both
weak and strong at different times and in different
areas. If weakness frightens you, you're still five years
old inside.

How close to Dr. Jekyll and Mr. Hyde is your personality? You may call it politic, diplomatic. Too many others might see it as two-faced, petty, and competitive.
When you're nice to someone's face or only in circumstances in which you wish to cover up your resentment and envy, do you feel good? When you go behind
their backs to undermine, distort, or damage, do you
feel better? Children in the throes of sibling rivalry
often behave this way. In their minds, there is only a
certain amount of love or attention available. They
figure that if someone else gets any at all, that automatically cuts down their share. As you grow from
childhood you normally come to understand that lovingness and acceptance are qualities of a person, and
not quantities to be doled out. If you are a Jekyll and
Hyde in your private and professional life, it's because
you fear, deeply fear, that someone else's having something—attention, success, ability—means you somehow are or will get less, so you greedily become a
person who enjoys little of what you have simply because others have.

Do you get bored easily? Some of you think that getting bored with things is a sign of your intellectual superiority. Some of you think that your boredom is a sign you're in the wrong place or with the wrong person. There are times when that's true. But if you've got a pattern of boredom rather than sporadic experiences with it, your boredom may be a signal of a growing depression where your sense of hopelessness disintegrates your interest in anything. Boredom is also an escape. If something is difficult for you to grasp, if you don't understand what's going on, if you're afraid to be found out in some negative way, you may call what you're feeling boredom. No one expects you to stay with anything that bores you, so now you have an easy way out of whatever is threatening you. Maybe no one else knows it, but you know it. And every time you flee, you further undermine your own sense of courage, strength, and ability, creating a need for more escape routes. Whatever it is, stay with it long enough to find out and work through whatever it is that makes you want to run.

You want to be liked and accepted, but what game do you play? Perhaps you are the flirt who capitalizes on charm and seduction. Maybe you're the scrooge who rejects everyone and everything first. Or the aggressive, love-me-or-leave-me loudmouth. It could be that you stand back and scrutinize everyone else—a real critic. The storyteller is interesting, for a while. The drunk anesthetizes his awareness altogether. The wallflower disappears into the woodwork. With these behaviors, you try to entice acceptance or deny your need of it. These disguises serve only to hide your real self. The act may be accepted, but you're still hidden. All that game playing is really to hide your true identity and vulnerability. If someone doesn't like you, or so you imagine, you can always say, "Well, that wasn't really me, anyway." Very cute, but very lonely.

Praise feels good; criticism hurts. So why do you listen so much more to the criticism? One woman got more hurt by her husband's comment when he was in a tantrum than she was soothed by his comments when he was in a loving mood. Why? You will be more sensitive to criticisms and anger when you are not sure of your own value, lovability, or desirability. It's a feeling of always looking over your shoulder to make sure no one finds out what you are really like. I'll prove it to you this way. Pinch your skin somewhere. It probably doesn't hurt much. Now pinch your skin where you already have a bruise. Now that hurts! It's the same with emotional pain. You hurt the most where you are already bruised. If your partner rages like an unchained demon, get annoyed and bored with it, and realize that if you get caught up in it, that's because you're buying what he's saying. It's not his fault. It's your unhealed wound.

Are you a martyr? Martyrdom is not a predicament. It's a design made for your life. Why would you choose to suffer like that? Perhaps your suffering provokes guilt and pity. Oh, that sounds so manipulative, and it is. Control over others is hard to give up. It gets you some things you want, like attention and caretaking. It tries to fend off some unpleasant things, like criticism and responsibility. But you pay a price for this. You have a sense of powerlessness, worthlessness, and hopelessness. You believe that there is no other way to get what you want or to be somebody. You believe that you may deserve the pain you live with. You believe that speaking directly about what you need and want is bad. You are afraid of deep, intimate contact with others. You must recognize that if you're suffering on and on with the same situation, it's because you're at home with it and afraid of leaving those few comforts.

Why work toward a specific destination when life seems to be a series of detours? A show-business friend of mine in a philosophical moment said he didn't know why he bothered with résumés, interviews, and agents. It seemed that all his best opportunities came out of left field, from people and places he either didn't know or never suspected. But you need motivation, direction, and accomplishment to feel satisfaction. That takes planning. And rather than become disappointed that the outcome isn't exactly what you planned, be amused and grateful for the opportunities you did get. Without your original plans, you wouldn't have gotten the exercise of trying and learning. Others wouldn't have gotten the opportunity to experience you. Working toward a goal, any goal, is minimally a way of keeping your engines revved for whatever turns out to be the trip you make.

Are you struggling for happiness? In a relationship, do you find yourself working uphill, trying to find the real person underneath your partner's withdrawal, alcoholism, violence, inconsistent behavior, or noncommunicativeness? Do you sometimes ask yourself, "Why do you work so hard?" Are these some of the excuses you placate yourself with: "When he's not being like that, he's really nice"; "Oh, I know she's difficult, but she needs me"; "But I love him"; or, "There really isn't much better out there." While it is true that building good relationships takes commitment, compromise, care, and consistency, perpetual struggling is a cue that you are someplace unhealthy for you and you're there because you don't feel confident, competent, and worthy. Here's a test: Imagine or examine someone really wonderful. Do you feel you deserve it? Do you worry that it won't last? Do you panic that something else terrible will happen to ruin everything? Then the real struggle is within yourself.

What are you waiting for? Many of you have gone through some terrible experiences: betrayal, abuse, sexual exploitation, psychological pummeling. And now it's as if your life were on hold waiting for some word from the perpetrator before you can move on and live your life. The obvious problem is that most people want to forget the terrible things they've done—forget to the point of denial and repression. They say to you, "What's past is done. I can't change it. Why don't you just go on and forget it?" But you can't; you fight them. For what? You're not sure. Are you waiting for an apology? If it comes, aren't you likely to say, "That isn't enough"? Are you waiting for them to die? If they do, don't those feelings remain? Are you waiting for them to make the past never have happened? You've got to rely on and respect your perception of what happened regardless of their position.

You've got to separate your guilts from the reality of your victimization. In other words, you need yourself more than you need anything from them.

Want to get *exactly* what you want? Forget it. You may be demanding all sorts of things from your loved ones and not getting much of what you're asking for. So you get to feeling deprived and victimized. To break the pattern, you try to get new loved ones. But the same thing keeps happening. The next place to look is inside yourself. For example, it's one thing to ask for attention and another to ask for a certain kind of attention at certain times of the day, given in a certain way. It's important to be clear about your wants and needs and innermost desires. But it's never rewarding to demand that the other person conform to your whole way of thinking about just how things ought to be done. Just as you feel a need to see your will expressed, so does everyone else. So learn to settle with their meeting your needs in ways that fit their own style, personality, and needs. If it has to be your way or not at all, it's probably going to be not at all. And that's a lousy compromise.

So how do you feel when people save you from your-self? Have you had people say to you, "Oh, I was going to tell you, but I didn't want to get you all upset"? They're clearly trying to be tuned in to your moods with sensitivity. That seems obvious. So why do you get so angry when they do that? It's that the underly-ing message sounds like, "You can't handle it." The attempt is being made not to overload your "cope-ability." There are times when that is appreciated, and then there are those other times when you feel belit-tled. What you need to do first is to think about how you do react or maybe overreact to things, frightening those close to you into being overprotective. This doesn't mean you have to stop ricocheting around the room if that's how you cope best with stress. But per-haps it would help to clarify for others that although you get angry or suffer, neither you nor the relation-ship will be mortally wounded by the truth.

There's an old saying about not being able to get blood out of a stone. You may be thinking of that old saying when you underestimate, understimulate, underchal-lenge yourself. Ever hear of second wind? It's a fasci-nating physiological response you get when you are exerting yourself physically. Just when it seems like you're heaving over the breaking point, you find your-self breathing easier, working with less effort. Have you given yourself the opportunity to find your psychological second wind? Just when you think you intellectually can't produce any more or emotionally survive any more, that's the point at which you may experience an extra surge of creativity or the energy to survive. It's too easy to talk yourself out of finding that point. You could excuse yourself with the other old saying, that enough is enough. Although that is the truth, it doesn't specifically designate your limits. Sometimes fate makes you stretch. Don't wait for that.

How do you survive a situation that is just no fun at all? I counsel many people who are going through unpleasant transitions in temporary job situations they hate, living somewhere they despise, being around people they loathe. It certainly can become a challenge to simple survival. I don't like simple survival. I think you should hope for and work toward more, even in the midst of misery. And there's always a way. Don't wait for your attitude to change before you change your behaviors. Count on changed behaviors having a wonderful effect on your attitude. Find the chuckle. That's right, find the chuckle. There always is one, you know. One woman I counseled was working in a depressing place with depressed people. She already had trouble with depression. We talked about finding the chuckle. She struggled with that until one day she came in elated. She had found the chuckle to get by at work. "What is it?" I asked all excited. "Well," she said, "I smile, laugh, and talk to everyone. The chuckle is me."

Having trouble making decisions because your feelings seem to jump around? Maybe you wait until you find yourself sufficiently angry, hurt, bored, or numb to make that gut-wrenching decision. And then the feeling passes and you respond by changing your mind. And so it goes again and again. After a while, you begin to feel stupid, even insane. Definitely embarrassed. You know, second thoughts are one thing; a change of mind based on new information, concrete reasons to persist, could be a wise move. However, if your decision making oscillates at a frequency approaching the speed of light, something's wrong. Could it be that you don't really mean the decision, that it is really an attempt for attention, power, manipulation? Or could it be that you don't realize that states of mind and heart pass, but resolutions made on the picture of the whole don't have to? Of course, there are fears and regrets and desperate wishes, and they pass too.

Do you always put your worst foot forward? You may think of putting your best foot forward as the only way to protect yourself against criticism and rejection. Yet some of you put your worst foot forward to do the very same thing. Think of the times you come on all gruff and testy so that a new person won't see your sensitive and vulnerable side. Or the times you come on cold and stern so that no one will think you're needy but frightened of intimacy. It could be that you're abrasive and rejecting so that you won't be unnerved by a sexual approach. It might be that you come on all weepy and needy in the hope that no one will ask of you what you fear you won't be able to do. Your worst foot forward might save you from confronting your immediate fear, but you end up not confronting too many nice things either. Instead of your best foot or your worst foot, your best bet is to put forth your real foot and learn to deal with your real and your imagined fears.

"Oh, she just likes to suffer. I think she enjoys being a martyr." In the years I have been counselor, I've never yet met anyone who enjoyed suffering. Yet I've met so many who desperately hang on to situations and behaviors that cause suffering. The most obvious question is "Why?" Examine your own life for the answer. How many times have you let something go on and on because it just seemed easier, safer, more familiar, or

simply the only way you thought things should be?
"Oh sure. But I'd never let myself suffer like that," you
say. That which is yours always seems more reasonable, more easily rationalized and explainable than
you so easily judge in others. It comes down to a matter of degree, because you all compromise, look away,
try to survive. Next time you see someone who you
think gets off on suffering, look again. You'll see a person who feels helpless, frightened, and frustrated.

I can't think of one good thing to say about disappointment. When you finally have a success, it's easy
to be generous and philosophical about what you've
gained from surviving all those disappointments. But
till then, disappointments are devastating. The worst
thing about disappointments is that you don't get what
you were counting on. The more you counted on it,
the bigger the disappointment. The more your whole
life has been in suspended animation, waiting for this
miracle, the more shattering the impact when it never
comes. The destructiveness of disappointments often
is based on your not accepting or realizing that there
are options other than those you've been counting on.
Life doesn't always cough up our dreams or our due.
But it always gives us alternatives. That's where our
courage and will to squeeze satisfaction out of life
come in. Are you ready to start seeing disappointments as opportunities?

Do you try to express feelings in such a way as to make you look like a good little boy or girl? Unfortunately, many of you discovered as children that when you expressed certain feelings, there was hell to pay. Maybe when you showed hurt, anger, indignation, or annoyance, your parents punished you in thought, word, or deed. Anything from "In this family, we always smile no matter what" to "Don't you make that angry face at me!" So you learned to tailor the outward expression of your emotional reactions to avoid their displeasure and to court their approval. And that wreaked havoc on your insides, didn't it? Are you still doing that? Maybe you're still behaving like the needy and dependent child, letting others edit your identity to fit their comfort. Perhaps you need to discover you can and have grown up. You can be and share the real you.

We all need a little luck now and then. Whether you look at it as circumstance, timing, whim, or accident, luck is an essential ingredient of good fortune. It's frustrating and infuriating, but you can't program, plan, or produce luck. So what can you do to survive the frustrations of trying, working hard, giving it your all, hanging in, when none of it seems to go your way? What you do to survive is dependent upon what that success means to you and how balanced your life is. Lots of you may be postponing living until your ship comes in. Others of you may be putting everything you have into that one end. You may see yourself as not having a life at all without that one success or event you're counting on. If you want to survive those chance misses of good fortune, stop postponing your life and start seeing yourself and your life as more than that success.

The biggest factor in your not being able to make choices is your lack of faith in yourself. One lady felt trapped. She didn't want a divorce. She wasn't sure how she would make out alone. She did not want to be close to her husband because of all his rotten behaviors. There was really no immediate solution to her bind. Both leaving and staying seemed unpleasant. The key was her lack of a sense of autonomy, strength, and self-esteem. Since she feared being alone, she didn't rock the boat too much. That meant she wouldn't ask, demand, complain, or work through her dissatisfactions with her husband, lest he get mad and leave her. That meant she had to "take it" to survive. She did that by withdrawing into her own world. When you are somewhere because the alternative seems too scary or difficult, you're not really choosing to stay. When you are somewhere not out of choice, you generally have resentment for being there. This all becomes a stalemate of a not-too-peaceful coexistence. The way out is to come to believe you can be a whole person unto yourself. Then you have choices.

Are you sometimes unsure of whether you're thinking one way or the other about something? "I'm not sure whether I'm being selfish or not, mean or not, wrong or not, bad or not." I admire you for considering the possibility that you could be naughty. But when you ask the "or" question, you make it impossible to answer. You are never that purely bad or good or right or wrong. The reality is that you are capable of experiencing a mixture of thoughts and feelings. If you demand of yourself only one feeling at a time, then you'll always feel guilty and confused by the real feelings you do have. Yes, it's possible to love someone and have negative feelings about him. Yes, it's possible to want something and have reservations. Yes, it's possible to feel you're right and still wonder. When you were a kid, that spanking told you when you were wrong or bad. As an adult, you know that some negative consequences don't necessarily mean you were wrong or bad. As an adult, you are your own weather vane of approval.

Do you realize how frustrated you really are? You go along each day, struggling with the annoyances, irritations, and furies your world always seems to have available, thinking, "I'm getting tired of this, you know." But for the most part, you feel you have yourself and your world under control. You seem to have little patience with the harmless quirks of your loved ones, though. Your dog's usually cute behaviors become bothersome. Your interest in other people's point of view vanishes as they become just another object to deal with. Even feeling sexy is a memory. Well, if that's you, you aren't handling your stresses well at all. You have given priority status to those things in your life that pain you. And in your pain, you have no place left for the more pleasurable aspects of your life. Stop it! Just stop! Imagine, for a moment, your life without the disappointments and frustrations. Isn't that nice? You do have all that available to you now, within your reach: hobbies, loving, playing, creating. Do it.

What does failure mean to you? When I say the word "failure," what's the first word that comes to your mind?

"Bad?" "Final?" "Unlovable?" "Unforgivable?" "Fear?" "Sadness?" "Punishment?" Whew! How negative and frightening! No wonder you hesitate to try something new. Why tempt those feelings? Louis Pasteur said that no experiments ever failed. No matter how they turned out, they told you something. You just needed to be willing to listen. How can you be willing or able to listen to the message of an apparent failure through that roar of negativity? You need a change in attitude first. Remember that the first scientist who wondered what was killing off the bacteria he was trying to grow discovered antibiotics. He was not the first person to notice this happening. He was just the first not to see it as a failure in the experiment. There's a lot to learn about yourself from the experience of so-called failures. So yearn for them.

# CHAPTER 8

# Anger Management

Are you rude? Admit it. Your flow of "Please, may I's" and "Thank you's" is down to a bare trickle. When you bump into someone, you give them a shove because they got in your way. A person who is doing something slowly because he is older, or young and trying, or not very experienced or bright, gets a helping fist from you instead of compassion. I'm sure that this isn't the way your folks brought you up. You were probably a nicely behaved little kid, so what's happened? Okay, now come the excuses. You know it's wrong to be rude, but you're so tired, so stressed, you just can't help it. Everyone seems to be a stranger, making you feel removed or alienated. And what's the point of being polite anyway, when everyone else is rude? An excuse by any other name still stinks. The "everyone" out there starts with you. You need to be the kind of person you think you should be, regardless of how others behave or how many slings and arrows of outrageous fortune use you for a pincushion. Are you listening? Good! And thank you.

Do you risk your life for a moment of feeling powerful? Ever saunter slowly across a pedestrian crosswalk, your body language shrieking a challenge? When the car in front signals to move into your lane, do you accelerate and close up the space? Do you cut people off when making turns? And when thwarted in such attempts, do you shout obscenities (or pantomime them)? If so, what's going on with you? You may feel that some of these acts are justified because of such and such, but the truth is, you are risking your life for a moment of glory. These acts are to get just anyone back for the frustrations, failures, and embarrassments you've suffered. And, in doing so, you heap frustrations onto strangers, priming them to release their anger haphazardly. This chain of social disregard and violence didn't begin with you, but it could end with you. When you're feeling low, you need a wave, not a fist, so smile.

Are you a spiteful person? If you're a spiteful person, you willfully injure or thwart another out of your own feelings of hurt and anger. Here are some examples: The person you think you love cares about another. Understandably you're hurt, so you make scary phone calls, put sugar in his car's gas tank, and undermine him at work. Or someone else has gotten the promotion or position you've been dying for. Do you start bad rumors about her? What's the end result? Does that person suddenly love you? Do you now get a better job? Are you happier? Are you better off? Surviving hurts and disappointments is difficult. Perhaps you use the technique of evening the score as a means of feeling powerful in the midst of painful hopelessness. Perhaps you do it in the hope that now someone else will understand the pain you've gone through, so he'll fix it for you. Spitefulness only digs your hole deeper, leaving you less loved, even by yourself.

Aware of being too impatient with yourself? Do you get an idea or get started on something and get on your own case immediately? Do you get irritated with yourself when it's obvious you need time for practice or execution? Do you berate yourself for not knowing how to do things before you even start? I'm certain you wouldn't dream of reacting that way to anyone else. Yet you are your own worst taskmaster. Impatience with yourself is your admission that you are no good. Surprised? You shouldn't be. Impatience says, "You're not smart enough, fast enough, creative enough." Impatience says, "You're not important. It's what you do that's important." Impatience robs you of certain pleasures: the pleasure of a leisurely discovery, the pleasure of the trial-and-error method of working something through, the pleasure of the process. Impatience with yourself betrays your need to perform rather than live. It makes your whole existence focus on the swallowing instead of the tasting.

Is there someone you still hate? One lady still hates the woman she found in her husband's arms during the last trimester of her own pregnancy. She and her husband have never talked about it much. A young man still hates his father for being an alcoholic who beat him up and argued a lot with his mother. Neither of those responses seems unreasonable considering the circumstances. What is unreasonable is the magnitude and duration of the reaction. The lady holds on to her anger at the other woman to distract herself from her greater pain, the reality that her husband, during their pregnancy, was having sex with someone else. If she had to face that, she might have to think of confrontation, and perhaps even divorce. If the young man doesn't focus all his hate on his father, he might have to deal with the reality that his mother did little to protect him, making him an emotional orphan. He might also have to face how much like his father he's becoming. What does the focusing of your hate keep blurred in your life?

Have you turned mean, nasty, and rude? Perhaps you're not mean, nasty, and rude with those close to you, but what are you like in public? Do you tell people to "drop dead" when they ask you not to smoke in a restaurant, an elevator, or another closed space? Do you speed up and block people off when they signal a lane change that could put them, oh my, in front of you? Do you stand in an elevator, apparently in a trance, while someone rushes toward the closing doors? Do you talk loudly in movie theaters and make threats when someone shushes you? Do you use hand signals implying commands of sexual contortions in response to being caught in the wrong? Does any of this make you feel any better? Improve your day? No, it probably doesn't. Keep in mind, also, that these are all acts of violence. Fists, guns, and knives aren't the only ways you have of brutalizing one another. Verbal and psychological abuses are just as deadly to your well-being, someone else's, and that of society as a whole.

Confrontation doesn't have to mean all-out war. Anger doesn't have to be expressed angrily. Confrontations don't have to be exercises in humiliation. It might be that you're angry, not because of what the other has done, but because of how you handled it. If someone does or says something that hurts or upsets you, disappoints or frustrates you, do you blow up instantly or simmer it all into a concoction of distorted fury? All in all, you're hurting yourself more than the other person's power to get to you. Have you tried checking it out? You know, making sure your perception is accurate. Have you tried thinking the whole thing through, looking at what you know and have experienced about that person, to decide whether they had some malevolent intent or were momentarily self-absorbed and thoughtless? As you can see, there is lots to talk about when you're angry with someone. Instant or delayed fury is not your only alternative. If you've thought it was, then you've got the notion that intimates are inherent enemies.

Does your control control you? I worked with one man in counseling who, after a hard day's work, somehow felt compelled to check things out, like the top of the refrigerator and the corners of bathrooms, to make sure his wife got everything as clean as it was supposed to be. Another man would lecture his wife at great length about the proper way to take care of things whenever he found that she left something out of place. Both men complained about having to keep

on their wives about this. Both men justified the necessity for their behaviors. Both men agreed that, on a
daily basis, the issues were truly small. Both couldn't
stop themselves. Their wives felt that these men were
controlling them. Actually, both of them were controlled by their own need to control. Control is one
way of quelling anxieties. If you are anxious about not
being perfect enough, successful enough, or sane
enough, having order and, more so, enforcing order in
others is a way you try to keep from becoming or even
feeling your own worst fears. Order on the outside is
important when you are trying to suppress emotional
chaos on the inside.

Why do you take out your anger on the ones you love?
You know those times when you're trying to fix something or maybe work out a problem in your head.
Things just aren't going well. You're getting edgy. Your
partner happens by, and you snap at him brutally. You
hate yourself afterwards, even as you try to make him
responsible for either your problem or your mood.
Part of that reaction on your part is shame or embarrassment. You simply don't like to have those closest
to you, from whom you need love and approval, see
you not at your best. If you don't know something or
can't do something, a tiny childlike voice inside you
says, "Oh-oh. I've failed. I might be spanked or abandoned." In defense of these fears, you attack, becom-

ing mean and nasty—just the kind of behavior for which you ought to be spanked. Part of your nasty reaction during those times of stress to your ego is also because your partner hasn't made an instant save of you. You become angry with your beloved for not rescuing you from your own bad feelings about yourself. Keep this in mind next time you blast out at your loved ones.

How easy is it for you to overlook other people's good points? Boy, we can count on you to be right on the mark, wary and waiting for others to show weakness, meanness, forgetfulness, insensitivity, disloyalty. You react with triumphant "ahas" and then lapse into your routine, cynical speech on the rottenness of people. How do you react when people don't fit that bill? When they're either benign and harmless or actively supportive and pleasant? Do you sigh a relief at this oasis of kindness? Or do you discount it all by saying, "It's probably an act; just wait, they'll show their true colors"? Unfortunately, there are just enough people doing and saying crummy things to justify your negativity. But nothing justifies your feeling hurt, angry, and defensive all the time. That's a miserable state for you to be in, regardless of how others behave. It's too big a drain on your well-being. Try being as attentive, aware, and responsive to the good points as to the bad points in people. This attitude might lower your anxiety and challenge them to be nicer.

How do you get something that's bugging you out of your mind? You know that frustration. Someone has upset or angered you. You were treated unfairly. That creep caused you problems. You can't seem to get it out of your mind. You try not to talk about it over and over again, yet you find yourself silently agonizing. You're distracted momentarily and then it seems as though you're pulling yourself back into those painful thoughts. What you're doing is distilling your whole existence down into that one problem area. Whether or not it will take some effort on your part to take care of the problem, the obsessive ruminating isn't helping you or those around you. Distractions that don't require substantial effort on your part might help. I exclude effort, because if you're frustrated by the distraction itself, you'll probably just compound those other feelings. Humor might work for you. Try saying to yourself something like, "I'm going home for dinner and I'm going to be fine, but that creep's still going to be dumb and ugly." It may sound somewhere between crass and useless, but it might work.

What's the best way to handle a rude person? It probably happens to you every day. You hold the door open for a stranger in a store and they waltz through it with the silence of bored royalty. You wait patiently in line at the supermarket and someone doesn't want to bother waiting on even the express line. So she boldly steps in front of you saying, "Do you mind if I go first? I just have these two little things." In all of these situations, you probably respond with constipated fury as you feel trapped into appeasement, lest you look impolite. Friends, there's a huge difference between retaliatory nasties and a display of your appropriate response to their cheekiness, gall, and general self-centeredness. So stand your ground, smile, and state the facts, such as, "Excuse me, I'm next on line. Please wait your turn." Stay firm, but don't lose that friendly edge. It makes you all the more formidable. If due respect isn't shown you, you show 'em how it's done.

Do last-minute changes and frustrations drive you crazy? You're sure you're living under a black cloud. For instance, you've taken care of your part but someone else hasn't taken care of hers, and that leaves you up the creek. That's enough to drive you into fury. You feel like punching or kicking something or someone. Like giving up. Tearing your hair out. You know what you've done? You've added self-insult to your own injuries. All of that behavior in response to the problem is self-destructive. You're punishing yourself for fate or other people's absentmindedness or stupidity. When you're reminded that you're overreacting, you probably get defensive and try to justify your fury based on what injury or frustration you've sustained—justified or not. By sustaining your furious, hysterical reaction, you sustain the original injury. Now rather than punishing yourself with fury, reward yourself with a little bit of humor.

I want you to tell me the last day you had when nothing went wrong. This is where coping comes in. Most people think that coping means not getting upset. That's wrong. Coping is an attitude. It keeps the slings and arrows of outrageous fortune from targeting in on a headache, an ulcer, a temper tantrum, and so on. Try this. First, list the numbers one through five. Second, next to each number, write down one of your typical reactions to frustrations with the number five next to your worst reaction. For example, for number one, you might write "laugh." For number three, you might put "complain for an hour," and for the big number five, "throw a fit." Now the next time an irritation of any size occurs, decide which number it belongs to by the kind of response you decide it should have. I'll bet you're already wondering why you would ever choose to go to number five at all. Now that's a good question.

What do you do when someone gets in the way of your best efforts? Before you decide how and to what magnitude to react, let's analyze the situation. For example, adversity doesn't always pulverize. Sometimes it energizes. What you are used to doing and what really may be your best effort may be surprisingly different. And it might just be that those irritations may serve as challenges, causing you to tap into creativity and energy you never realized you had—in which case, you may be grateful for the intrusion. Second, and again before you react, do consider whether it is another person's intent to hurt you or whether the annoyance to you is merely a by-product of his insecurities, like when someone's trying too hard. You have a right to feel any emotions you do feel, including anger, resentment, and frustration. How you handle this should depend not on how you feel about what happened, but on what you analyze the situation to be—or you might hate yourself later.

Doesn't it just drive you crazy when people say to you, "Don't get so upset, it doesn't help"? It's enough to make you scream. There you are, hurt, upset, frenzied, and furious. You're the one who's been wronged by a friend or fate. You're the one who has to sustain the loss, pain, or embarrassment. Now, to top it all off, you have to be told that being upset doesn't help. You remember hearing a psychologist on some TV show telling you how you should get your anger out so you won't get ulcers, headaches, or skin rashes. You use that now as your permission to rant and rave. And what do you find out? That indeed, it doesn't help. Hurt and anger acted out like some temper tantrum is dangerous. It is stressful to you physically. You might say or do something regrettable. Your intimates may become bruised. Use your anger to motivate you toward more constructive behavior such as changing in the way you handle certain people or situations. Or work on becoming more philosophical about your emotional investment in some of your activities.

Doesn't being rude, selfish, troublesome, or mean make you feel bad or at least embarrassed? I'm worried that some mutation might have caused too many of us all to lose that essential part of our civilized being, a conscience. Notice how many times you can cut people off in traffic, cut ahead of people in lines, neglect amenities, offend and abuse others in public, and, in general, show hostile disregard for the rights and sensitivities of others. Sociologists talk about the stress of the economy, racial tensions, and crowding. Psychologists talk about the breakup of the family and the religious influence. I am talking to you about your responsibility for your behavior. Those of you unhappy inside yourselves, about yourselves, may not realize your punitive potential. You may find all sorts of excuses to scapegoat innocent strangers, yet the truth may be simply that you hurt and, therefore, you don't care if you hurt others.

Are you punishing yourself for past decisions? I was counseling a thirty-five-year-old woman and her mother. The daughter was complaining about not getting enough loving attention when she was growing up. The mother described the rages the father would get into when she showed her children attention or affection. She explained being the kind of woman who just listened to her husband to keep the peace. The mother has since divorced that abusive and alcoholic father. He would never get any help. Now she regrets that she was so acquiescent all those years, holding back her feelings and opinions. The mother asked me if it would have been better for everyone if she had confronted the father and fought it out each time he was in a rage. It occurred to me that the man might have become homicidal and that it might have been the mother's peacemaking that kept the family whole and safe as long as it was. It's too simple to say what should have happened. It's much more difficult and compassionate to explore what was good in the intent.

Lose your temper too often with your kids or pets? If you are losing your temper and patience too often with your puppy or child, you are missing an opportunity to have things the way you want them. A little boy in a restaurant began to cry. His mother shook him vigorously screaming, "What are you crying about?" The crying got louder. Riding her bike, a lady had a Doberman puppy on a leash. The puppy got frightened at the bark of another dog and got tangled up in the leash. Of course, the lady fell off the bike, screaming at the dog to calm down. The point of these stories is that both these people lost patience and neither got what they wanted, a calmer child or pet. If you really want what you want, go after it. That means give the situation what it needs for both of you to get your goodies. Both women needed to soothe and reassure their wards. That took staying patient. So the key to getting what you want is not coming unglued at the loss of it but patiently, seducing it back.

What do you do when someone is so rude to you that you feel like you're going to lose your control? It probably happens too often. People talk in the movie theater and get obnoxious when you politely ask then to sssshhhh. People endanger your life in traffic and get threatening when you honk or yell in frightened anger. On the telephone, in stores, in the street, you find yourself in situations where people totally ignore the basic notions of civilized social behavior. At first you're stunned; then their persistence at rudeness gets you angry. If you start yelling at them, they'll only escalate. When you lose your cool, they feel vindicated in their behavior. After all, how else do you behave with a screaming mimi? I'm not telling you to be a goody two-shoes or a revolving cheek. With quiet firmness say, "Please go to your place in line." If they keep a-comin', either get someone in charge or back off and preserve your blood pressure, stomach, and peace of mind.

Do you become part of the problem or part of the solution? I saw a car stall out at a corner. There was a long line of people waiting to make right-hand turns at that corner, they were honking and yelling, threatening, complaining, pounding on their steering wheels, and generally carrying on. That poor fellow in the stalled car was frightened, exhausted, frustrated, and feeling totally helpless. He gallantly tried to push his car himself, but he couldn't get it to move. I guess all of those impatient people believed this fellow either liked being stalled or had done it intentionally just to ruin their day. Why else would they yell at him so viciously? The man in the car behind the stalled vehicle stopped yelling and started thinking. I saw him smile, get out of his car, and help push the other fellow in this car to the side of the road. Then other passersby joined in to being part of the solution to this problem. What would you have done?

Do you go to war too easily? Maybe you've had a little fender-bender. It could be that the person in line with you is also running late. Perhaps the clerk is doing his best. Do you see most everyone in the world as an impediment to your progress and welfare? On a day when everything seems to be going wrong, it's easy to feel that way. Rationally, you know it's not true, but you can create that environment by your attitude. If in asking for assistance, in waiting, in trying to get somewhere, you display impatience, annoyance, disrespect, and anger, you are slapping the face of everyone else with a white glove and so the duel begins. Try approaching these people giving them the feeling that you need them. For example, "I've called so many extensions and keep getting different numbers to call. I feel lost and demoralized. Can you rescue me?" That person is going to be more willing to change the course of events in your day for the better. Try it.

Forget the best way. What's any way to deal with obnoxiousness? You're with someone who is becoming loud and rude in public. You're trying to deal with someone who is blatantly selfish or thoughtless. Other than get embarrassed, frustrated, and angry, what do you do? A major factor in your difficulty dealing with an obnoxious person is that his behavior breaks all the rules you live by. You simply can't imagine or easily accept that anyone could behave that way. Your response is to do whatever it takes to make this awful situation not exist. So you try to ignore it, apologize for it, calm it down, change it, all in an attempt to make reason and sensitivity out of something that is unreasonable and insensitive. As a one-shot deal, any one of those responses is fine. But if the situation is continual, your efforts will get you nowhere. When faced with obnoxiousness, do just that. Face it. Not with escalating hostility. Face it with directness, preferably laced with humor.

Sometimes retreat is the better part of valor. There always will be challenges to your better judgment or behavior. On the freeway, in a crowded store, at work, and even in the sanctity of home, people will consciously, unconsciously, or accidentally challenge you to a duel of primitive reactions such as one-upsmanship or revenge. Even the nicest of you might find yourself ripe for action if you're overly tired or your cope-ability is spent. The urge to act like Clint Eastwood for only a moment becomes tantalizing. You remember old cowboy movies where people were driven to respond to ridiculous challenges because they were called yellow. You want to show your stuff. You coil up, ready to strike. Think of the expenditure of negative energy. Think of how little difference there appears to be between your behavior and theirs. Think of how you could get hurt. Think of how you could hurt someone else. Maybe just pass it by.

What's the point of having enemies? Sometimes being designated an enemy by someone else is out of your control. Sometimes you push right into a circumstance of making or maintaining an enemy. That takes effort, planning, parrying. It may seem necessary in the beginning for whatever hurt or vengeful feelings you've experienced. In the long run, though, you may find that it is emotionally and psychologically expensive. There is another way. Put all people in categories. Have at the top category all those people you really love. Give them lots of intensity and energy. Have at the bottom category all those people you've decided to hate. Give them no intensity, no energy. It's bad enough they've done you wrong; don't give them the power to continually sap your energy. Besides, maintained energies can be dangerous at times and places you never anticipated. Escalation won't help you with what has been damaged. Perhaps your best revenge is simply not caring enough to send the very worst.

Should you stifle your anger? I'm all for open, honest communication. I just think you've got to be a good director and editor of your anger, or else a good casting agent, because people are going to be in and out of your life in great numbers if you aren't. How does being your own good director help you communicate? Well, timing, location, and mood are important. When others are busy, already frenzied or tired; or in the midst of dinner, a warm bath, or bedtime snuggling, these are not good moments to deal with heavy-duty and perhaps unpleasant argumentative issues. How does being your own good editor help you communicate? Bringing up the past, pulling in irrelevant guilt-provoking issues, unleashing the full range of your piled-up inner emotion, do not present your case in a way that anyone wants to listen to. If you want to be heard, heeded, or responded to, you've got to present your case with respect or the magnitude of your emotional and verbal assault will be reflected back in triplicate.

Now, I don't want to upset you, but aren't you just a little bit too touchy for your own peace of mind? Frankly, I don't care if you are right or wrong in assessing someone else's behavior as warranting an angry response or not. That's not the point. What is the point is that you spend too much time suffering from feeling offended, hurt, criticized, betrayed, or attacked. That means the serenity of your work, your rest, your fun is too frequently punctuated with warning sirens requiring you to mobilize defenses. The bottom line is how much time you spend feeling lousy and how much energy is expended in maintaining a defensive posture. Would you be willing to try something different? I'm not sure what it'll be. You've got to decide that for yourself. The very next time you start feeling touchy, do something new. It might be to ask questions, get funny, say nothing, talk to someone about it—just do something new.

How do you cope with neighbors who are unfriendly, uncooperative, rude, and disrespectful? The first thing to remember in this situation is that if you are planning to give back nasty for nasty, you are probably outclassed by people who have had much experience in this kind of war, so forget it. Besides, if you retaliate in any way, you will simply be giving them proof of their need to be nasty. It might just be, however, that they have misunderstood some of your behaviors and intentions. Listen to their complaints. Don't argue each one. Give them their perceptions and promise to try better. This might bring down their anxiety. Next, model good-neighbor behavior as best you can, trying to be consistent until they stop seeing you as the enemy. If none of this works, you may be living next to people who are unstable and unreachable. You might need to minimize contact. If worst comes to worst, move.

When someone changes the ground rules on you or challenges you, do you respond with rage? Do you say things like, "How dare they do that?" Or, "Those stupid people are incompetent and just drive me crazy"? There is always some validity to your assessment of your situation and the people in it. But your rage response is more destructive to you than reconstructive of a more tolerable circumstance. Your rage response is meant to destroy the threat to your emotional or physical self. It's a defense mechanism that gets in gear automatically when you feel threatened with hurt or you feel helpless. There are instances when your rage will keep the dragons at bay. But it doesn't make you feel safer or more competent inside. Nor does your rage response endear you to others. If you feel frustrated, confused, or helpless, deal with those feelings, and don't let them turn into rage.

What does it mean to hate? Hate is a powerful emotion and physical reaction. On the physical side, I think of gritted teeth and clenched fists, protruding neck veins, high blood pressure, bulging eyeballs. On the emotional side, I think of helplessness, fear, denial, and blaming. What do they have to do with anger? One lady continued a relationship with a fellow for five years through his many affairs and general crummy treatment, all of which she knew about. She always found reasons to forgive and go back. Finally, her fantasy became threadbare and there was nothing for her to hold on to any longer. She became enraged with him all the time. In a way, her anger with him was unfair. She always knew his behaviors. He was consistent. And she had accepted them to continue the relationship. Her anger at him was really about herself or her sense of herself as too weak and frightened to deal with him better and to be in a better kind of relationship. Many times your anger toward others represents feelings toward yourself that you're trying not to face.

Let's hear it for revenge! You applaud, jump, and hurrah when the bad guy in the movies gets his just deserts, don't you? When someone digs a hole for you and falls into it, that's poetic justice. It's just great when evil swallows its own venom. But in real life, that doesn't happen as often as you'd like, does it? Now the problem with getting revenge is that it's not always possible, practical, or pleasant to arrange. Oh yes, you also have to consider looking bad yourself, and the possibility of retaliation. It's all so much cleaner and clearer in the movies. You may not dare to get your revenge on your original target for fear of reprisals, but you may not realize how that vengeful energy does get expressed. You may set yourself up for illness, injury, or failure. You may wreak emotional havoc upon those with whom you feel safer, usually family, pets, salespeople, neighbors, and inanimate objects. Everyone pays but the original bad guy. And oh yes, you've become a bad guy.

# CHAPTER 9

# *Ethics*

How do you know if you're doing the right thing? Doing the right thing: that's a tough one. It seems that no matter how you figure it, someone will be inconvenienced, disappointed, or hurt. When you try to figure it all out on some ethical or moral basis, it seems that something practical or expedient gets left out, and that complicates it. Don't bother going to ten other people for the answer. What you will get is ten perspectives. Good for helping you with your internal debate, but lacking one important factor: responsibility. Since others do not have that final responsibility, they can offer food for thought, but the answer carries responsibility. That's where you come in. When it comes down to it, every choice you make has a price tag attached. It may be that the reason you're having so much trouble making the decision is that you're trying to find one without a price to pay. There is no such answer. You must face which price you are willing to pay.

Why are you the bringer of bad news? Ever notice how you always seem to be the one to carry bad news to the person you say you love or admire? Maybe it's a family member, boss, teacher, or friend. You are the one to tell them what others are saying bad about them. You explain that you just want to keep them aware, and that no matter what anybody says, you are behind them. A pattern of bringing upsetting, perhaps not very useful, and definitely unsolicited bad news has intent. Here are the possibilities. It might be that you have jealous, resentful feelings toward this person. You may be unwilling to admit the feelings to yourself and deal with them directly, so you secretly punish that person by flinging other people's arrows. It may be that you want to feel special to that person. You tell them the terrible words of others, contrasting those with your feelings in the hope of being made special. The bottom line is that you're hurting, not helping, and fast becoming unpopular with that special person. Examine your motives and feelings.

How much would it take for you to sell out? When you sell out, you sacrifice your values, your honor, and your loyalty because you fear the loss of something more central to your being. As a kid, did you join the crowd in taunting an outsider or doing something else you believed to be wrong because you feared if you didn't you'd get thrown out of the group? Have you ever denied or forsaken your beliefs, your origins, your family or friends? These are all sellouts. There are so many ways to rationalize them. You could say there is no benefit to holding out because someone else will just benefit. You could say that it's a short-term sellout for a long-term potential benefit. You could say that there's no point to nobility; it just isn't valued much anymore. You could say it's just not practical to act on the basis of intangible ideas in a toughly tangible world. You could say any and all of that, and you may be right if you say that the only ones who really care if you do the right thing are you and a few others who are usually without clout. Well? Why isn't that enough?

How dark are your little white lies? I'm in favor of certain kinds of lying, like when telling someone the complete truth will serve only to hurt them. So you tell your child how incredibly wonderful that first recital was, or you tell your spouse that all-day cooking effort was a great success. Most of your lying may not be so considerate. Do you lie to save your own skin? In doing so, you probably don't realize how your credibility is being eroded by the corrosive effects of your inconsistent, hard-to-believe behavior. Do you lie for personal gain? This usually happens at work where you figure it's smarter to give people in power what you think they want. This may work for you until your self-esteem and their respect dwindle. Maybe you lie because you don't trust people to deal with you fairly and caringly when you are that frank and open. Then you lose twice: once for the betrayals you've had, and again for the perpetual need to hide your truths. If your lies are more to protect you than others, remember that you lose yourself in your lies.

Is your motto "Ask not what I can do for you until I find out what you can do for me"? Does your demeanor change when you're in the presence of someone who can do something for you, be it business or pleasure? Otherwise, you find yourself impatient, irritable, and even rude. You may not like having to kiss keisters like you do, even though it might be expedient and politic. That annoyance might be what you take out on strangers. Don't forget that your guts are in the middle. You are either being false or frenzied. That's the quickest way to emotional and physical upsets. Now, it is important to play certain games. It's expected and absolutely necessary, but when it comes to your whole life, when you become absorbed in the games, you lose out. There must be a balance between taking care of business and being at peace with yourself.

Are you afraid to tell the truth? You get in more trouble trying to say everything but the truth, don't you? By lying, distorting, or withholding, you say you're trying to protect others from hurt feelings. In the short run, I'll accept that. However, if your short-term protection only turns to oozing, growing resentment, then it's just no good for you or them. In that case, time just allowed the benevolent withholding of truth to evolve into a monster. Maybe it's better to reveal the truth up front, and allow everybody to experience whatever feelings they do, and you accept the consequences. Work toward everyone growing from that depth of passion evoked. Do you get choked up on the word "consequences"? It might be that your reason for withholding truth has to do with avoiding consequences. Telling the truth also has consequences. Dealing openly and honestly, though, gives the consequences more purpose, meaning, and direction. It's been said that the truth hurts. I think more often, the lie hurts more.

Why is it that evil seems to have so much power? You may be frustrated to death with injustices you've experienced or heard about. Unlike the happy endings of adventure stories, the good guys don't always come out ahead. As unfair and horrible as that may seem, it's a reality of life. Does it make you feel like giving up? Have you said, "If you can't beat 'em, join 'em," only to end up disgusted with yourself? There is another way. You can't control the world. You can't control people, but you can build something for yourself that is filled with more of the positive things in life than you see around you. Some people do that by their careful selection of friends. Others move to an area that displays more beauty. Many build families of love and loyalty. People give of themselves to people, creatures, and causes that allow them to feel like a positive participant in the happiness of others. You don't like things about the world? You can create a mini-world around you. Fill it well.

Should you always do unto others as you would have others do unto you? The "doing unto others" rule suggests that you treat other people with the same courtesy, respect, and fairness you would enjoy. However, there are at least two ways in which you may take that too far. The adage does not imply that you and others are exactly the same in tastes, needs, or responses to things. There are times when you give gifts, plan surprises, or make plans for others based on *your* interests rather than *their* pleasures. If it's also true that it's the thought that counts, your main thought ought to be about their preferences, even when they're different from yours. You also may treat others assuming that they have the same emotional responses you do—for instance, withholding the direct truth for fear they'd just collapse. Maybe that's your assumption based upon what you know about yourself. That's a time to respect their individuality and let them handle the situation in their own way. Besides, you might even learn something.

Now, what's the big deal about differences? Are you arguing a lot because someone has a different philosophy, opinion, or belief? Do you know why you're doing that? You may be thinking in an exclusionary way. That means if one thing is right or good, it's because it's the only thing which is right or good. If that's the way you feel (or is it "fear"?), then you will spend too much time unnecessarily justifying your position on the graves of other people's feelings or thoughts. It may be that you are overestimating the meaning and power of the obvious, like a label. Someone with an entirely different label like "Christian" or "female" or "senior citizen" or "handicapped" might not differ from you much at all in the basics of feeling or living. The word "difference" is simply an observation, not a threat or a value judgment. You could save yourself a lot of discomfort, avoidance, and argument if you looked into the substance of the person or situation for that which would please, satisfy, or stimulate you.

The other day, while I was waiting outside a store for opening time, a lady drove up in a pickup truck, by-passed at least twenty open spaces, and zoomed right into a handicapped parking spot. When she got out, I said, ever so gently, "Perhaps you didn't notice that this is a handicapped parking space?" She didn't bother to look back as she said, "So go tell someone." Astounded, I came back with, "I did. I told you." She ignored me. I had naughty fantasies of letting the air our of her tires to pay her back. Even though I felt justified in defense of a principle, something wouldn't let me do it. Call it conscience or guilt or that my mother was with me. Watching her disregard for social rules and feeling totally helpless to change her, stop her, or get back at her got me so frustrated, it took me an hour to calm down. When you act with flagrant, selfish disregard, you are powerful at the moment. Is that what you're needing? A sense of supremacy? And if you saw your children doing the same thing, would you feel proud of the dynasty you'd created?

Does placing the blame, even if correctly, really help? Indeed, pointing an honest finger that keeps you out of the pokey will definitely help. Yet there are times when placing blame, even correctly, doesn't add much to your well-being. A lot of you grow up, feel troubled and go into therapy, or read a self-help book and get the notion that the reason you're in trouble today is because your parents messed you up yesterday. A popular idea is that a confrontation with them expressing outrage, resentment, and disappointment is a creatively therapeutic exorcism. My experience as a therapist is that it is usually painful and destructive, and it generally doesn't magically eliminate all current demons of immaturity, insecurity, and incompetency. It is more useful to find a way of thinking or dealing with those who are to blame in a way that more directly helps you improve your life and your well-being. Dwelling on the contribution of those to blame is a quicksand trap, mostly for you.

Feel guilty saying you like to relax? Just look at how many of you feel guilt for saying you like kicking back and watching some TV or that you can take a whole weekend or more to just be a veggie. Maybe you can't even admit it to yourself. Radio listening or watching television can be restful, entertaining, informative. Doing nothing can be restful, entertaining, and informative too. Accept that the source of wonder is responding to your environment. Maybe noticing it, appreciating it for the first time. So don't feel you have to say, "Oh, I never watch TV I was just sick." Or, "My kid was watching it." And don't feel you have to say, "I had a good rest, but of course, I'd be bored to death to kick back for more than forty-eight hours." The world is not your vigilant, strict parent. The world is a place with lots of possibilities, and only you live with the inner awareness of your choices. Pseudointellectualism and excessive work ethic aside, you are not a worker bee or a machine. You are a person. Take some time to understand that potential.

Do you care about doing what's right? A friend of mine was pulling together some last-minute information for a television piece on "whatever-of-the-month clubs." She asked me if I knew whether parents are responsible financially if their children order from one of these clubs. I said I didn't know the law. But gee, why is that the most important question? Are you more concerned about how to get out of something legally than what you should do to take care of it morally? Justice is too often defined as the sum total of legal loopholes jumped through. The art of winning is seen as more important than being in the right or wrong. My answer to my friend was that if the parents did not make good on the bills, they were teaching their children the fine art of cheating. I'd have the kids work off the expenses, including mailing and handling. Even if it costs you money, effort, and a lot of embarrassment, it's easier to live with doing what's right.

You've heard a rumor concerning your friend. You know it will hurt your friend. What do you do? Nah, don't get involved. It will only backfire on you. What if the rumor isn't true? Look at the damage you've done then. It's none of your business anyway. You know, I can't really argue with these warnings. They may all be valid in some cases. Because that's true, there isn't any rule of thumb for handling this kind of predicament. Yet I would suggest you ask yourself these questions. And on the basis of your answers, you make your own decision. Here they are: Are you gloating inside about the rumor's content? Are you hoping to destroy a relationship between your friend and someone else? Are you wanting to appear the hero? Do you stand to gain by your friend's emotionally precipitant behavior? If the answers are all "no," and you feel your friend will be in a better position with the knowledge, then tell with loving support.

Do you respect your own opinions and decisions? Do you go back and forth with decisions? After you make a decision, do you spend your time arguing, defending, or rebelling against parents, teachers, friends, even your therapist? If so, then it is as though you think two important things are true: (a) there is always a clear and clean right decision; (b) everyone but you knows what that is. Both of those notions are false. Every choice made has benefits and losses. The question for you is which combinations of benefits and losses you are willing to live with. Since you are the one to walk the path chosen, others cannot possibly know best. They can offer challenges to your thinking, or more ideas for your repertoire. That doesn't make them smarter or right. It just makes them a potential help. The "right" decision is the one you respect yourself for making with consideration for your relationships, your welfare, and your future.

Want to motivate people to do the right thing? Most of your life, you may have experienced people attempting to motivate you by telling you what's wrong with the way you are or the way you do things. Was your first feeling one of motivation to change? Probably not. You more likely felt resentment and hostility and moved into a defensive stubbornness. Try motivating others by defining their behaviors in the positive, even if you feel you're stretching reality. After all, if it's kind and it works, why not? When your teenager always seems to forget to give you the where, when, and with-whom details, instead of telling her how irresponsible and rotten she's being, say something like, "I know you want to show me that I brought you up to be confident and careful so that I don't have to waste time worrying and watching. I appreciate that. It's just that sometimes I need to reach you with urgent messages and it would help if I knew where to find you." See how quickly you get cooperation redefining things in the positive, taking challenge and defensiveness out of the cycle.

What do you think telling the truth is really about? Telling the truth is generally taken to mean snitching on yourself, telling the bad things you've done. That's a grim proposition. I think telling the truth is essential to a good relationship. But the truth includes bigger things than turning yourself in. When you need a hug, tell the truth. When you're afraid and need support, tell the truth. When you have what you think are unacceptable thoughts or feelings, tell the truth. When you are happy or unhappy, tell the truth. For most of you, it may seem more difficult to contemplate such candor than to tattle on yourself. Yet that candor is life's breath to intimacy. Such truths define you, so you can become known, cared for, and responded to properly, something I know you'd like but feel uncomfortable doing. You've gotten through discomfort before. For these rewards, risk it.

Are you willing to consider the possibility that you're wrong? I realize that contemplating being wrong is uncomfortable. You don't like to look bad or stupid. So there's already a lot of resistance built into the system. But hang in there. I'll bet you could possibly enjoy being wrong about certain things. Consider your beliefs. One might be that things can't get better, or, "I'm stuck with the cards I was dealt," as one woman put it. Another belief might be that you don't really deserve love, or, "I back off from affection because I don't feel comfortable being treated well," as one man put it. These belief systems can pretty much limit your possibilities and flexibilities for joy, experimentation, and change. Yet you hang on to them for dear life. The problem is that you are treating your belief systems as though they were the truth or reality. Maybe you're wrong. Things can get better. You do have the right to happiness.

I know, I know! You just categorically won't even think of playing someone else's game, no matter what. You feel it is demeaning and irritating to be nice to someone you don't like or respect. You don't want to be in a situation that makes you feel as though you're stuffing your pride. So you get pouty, adamant, or righteous. You end up out. And they still have all the cards. There are times when you need to be practical. If you need the favors of little people with little egos who demand outsized offerings, think about it before you react. Would it really require you to scrap all your principles for all time? Would the results follow you around forever? Would you really be doing something against your whole moral fiber? If the answer is "no," if it's just a minor, insignificant display of what could be seen as incredible patience, tolerance, understanding, calm, or even humor, then do it, if it gets you what is important to you. Don't cut off your nose to spite someone else's face.

Why should you do what's right when you really don't want to? You have a lot of freedom. You live in a society that tolerates and protects a wide range of individual expression. There's an excitement in that. You don't always do what you should. What for? You don't want to wait your turn in line or forgo your conversation in a movie theater. You don't want to hold the door for the person behind you or speak politely. Why bother? You can do whatever you want, right? Well, freedom is a delicate balance. We all teeter between getting our own fulfillment and getting in the way of others trying to do the very same thing. That may not bother you so much. Who cares about the "them" out there? You don't even know them. There's a contagion in that thinking. Remember that they consider you the great unknown "them," too. The best way to protect yourself is to reinforce basic rules of courtesy and respect. That which excludes no one, always includes you.

Admit it! You lie. You lie for all sorts of reasons. To get yourself out of trouble. To create a situation beneficial only to you. To give a more appealing impression of yourself. Or because you're not sure what the truth is anymore. Lying is harder on you than anyone else. When you lie a lot, you have to stay vigilant, attentive, careful, lest you slip up. You suffer humiliation and punishment when your lying backfires. All in all, there is little peace. You probably think that lying has gotten you into and out of situations you would not have been able to maneuver successfully by any other means. Maybe so, but you're cheating yourself. You haven't learned how to use and how to trust more up-front, honest, vulnerable means of communication. In lying, you don't only manipulate others, you stifle your own growth. Honestly.

What should you do when you feel like giving up? There are times when giving up is the best thing to so. "Never give up!" sounds admirably gung ho, but there does come a point where the price is too big to pay a moment longer. The problem is that if you feel that way and act on it impulsively, you may regret it. So the key to separating inappropriate quitting from a timely giving-it-up may take some help from your friends. The guilt you experience in deciding to throw in the towel comes from a cultural tradition which demands you go down with the ship. All clichés aside, that's okay in the movies, but in your real life there are many issues to be considered in addition to stick-to-it-iveness, such as the effect your stubborn efforts are having on your loved ones, your health, your work, and your state of mind. It's good for you to know, to believe, that in giving up some activity, you are doing something good. If you are quitting in a frenzy of punishing spitefulness toward others or yourself, the guilt and regrets will plague you. There are those times when giving up will allow you to better live it up.

# CHAPTER 10

# *Sexual Relations*

Do you feel guilty about the fantasies you have while making love to your partner? Do you daydream about other partners or about what you think are naughty sexual acts in order to get aroused with your dearly beloved? Does it worry you that you do this? Do you think it means you're perverted or not in love with your partner? If so, you're being unfair to yourself. When our lives and relationships become comfortable, secure, and familiar, we're happy, content, but there is a danger in this comfort. The known and expected are generally not exciting, and enjoyable sex needs excitement. Some people bring the element of excitement back into their lives with affairs, drugs, swinging—behaviors which threaten the security that was the relationship. Your fantasies are a way to bring that excitement into your sexual relationship without threatening its existence. They may even give you some ideas on how to spice up your all-too-familiar sexual repertoire. So let your mind wander. Fantasize all you'd like.

How do you let go after a divorce? Whether or not you were the one to decide to leave, the ending of a long-term relationship is generally more difficult and painful than anticipated. The familiar, the comfortable are gone. New habits and arrangements have to be made for everything—sleeping, eating, socializing, living. Sometimes it isn't the person we want back so much as the return of the things they were, for the comfort, maybe even the safety they brought. Establishing a new life and identity is scary, challenging, disappointing, thrilling, and difficult. It's easy for you to get angry with your partner. If they'd only been different, you wouldn't have to be in this predicament. Letting go means moving on. When the moving on gets difficult, you resort to memories, nostalgia, regrets, and longing for what now seems like not such a bad alternative. Maybe you could and should go back. Maybe you could but shouldn't. Appraise your situation carefully before you rebound either back or forward. How does one let go after a divorce? Slowly, painfully, carefully.

Do you always know just what your dearly beloved is going to say or do? There is something to be said for predictability. It provides security because you know what to expect and what is expected. On the other hand, it is stagnating and boring. If your partner is so predictable, chances are that you are doing two things: being predictable yourself and working harder than you realize to keep them as predictable as they are. Have you been heard to say, "Oh, I'd travel more or take classes or some sport, but you know my beloved; he just won't go for it. He'll say . . ." In this case, you're using your partner as a shield against life and its risks and challenges. Keeping him staid keeps you safe, so you complain, but not quite enough to force a change. Another aspect of your perpetually proclaiming your partner's predictability is your unwillingness to see them change and grow. By telling them you know exactly what they'll do and say, you're telling them that who they have been, they will always be. If they change and grow, do you fear you will lose them?

Are you hopelessly stuck in a rotten situation? Do you and your beloved fight over the same issues? Important or not, nothing is resolved. It gets quiet—until the next time you fight it all over again. You recognize this—even feel frustrated with it—but nothing changes. Think of this behavior as a ritual that has symbolic meaning. The fight may serve to keep you both from getting too intimate for comfort. Is closeness scary to you? The fight may be the way you both try to show strength when other things in your life have undermined your self-esteem. Do you yell at or demean your partner to regain a sense of power or importance? You get the idea. Your being stuck is more than just an annoying circumstance. It has meaning. It means that you are not aware of some of your own feelings or are not being honest about them to your partner. You're not stuck in a situation. You are stuck inside yourself.

You're wasting your time if you're spending any of it trying to change yourself into what you think the opposite sex wants or values. How can you ever really know what the entire opposite sex thinks, needs, or wants? You'd have to condense the entire opposite sex into one individual, with one idea about masculinity, femininity, sexiness, or lovability. But you know everyone is different, so that really doesn't make any sense. Besides, this is all backwards. What happiness can you expect, trying to make yourself into something you're not just to get someone else to like you? Maybe you've done this already, only to discover that it left you frustrated, empty, feeling phony and even worse about yourself than when you started out. I have a suggestion. Stop working backwards. Look to yourself for your model of who to be, and polish it up the best you can. Then look for someone who has the sense to value you as you are.

Are you envious of the one you love? One man I counseled with his wife was always bugging her about her too-sexy clothes, flashy jewelry, and suspiciously outgoing personality. When we got down to talking about what attracted him to her in the first place, he admitted that her appearance and manner had a lot to do with it. And no, she hasn't really changed anything. What attracts you and what you can live with may be different. Why? What your emotions, needs, and passions respond to positively may shock and frighten your mind. That mind might be full of warnings and lessons about what is the right or the proper way. That confusion between your feelings and those old lessons may lead you to deny those feelings by punishing the naughtiness which attracted you. Next time you tell your partner that you resent the way they dress or act, ask yourself, and answer honestly: "Do I wish I could go and join them?" If the answer is "Yes, but . . . ," then the "but" part, not your partner, is the source of your problem.

What's the best way to be sexy? When you think of sexy, do you think first of perfume, slinky clothes, erotic come-ons, overt sexual behaviors? They may be part of the package, but many unhandsome, unadorned people throughout history have nonetheless been considered sexy. A lot of your sexuality comes from areas of yourself that can't be touched or primped. Your self-confidence, for example. Your level of comfort with your sensuality, too. Those give you a combination of power and vulnerability—an exciting mix. Your confidence and sensual comfort are increased with experience and self-acceptance. Nothing that can be bought, no potion to apply. Remember, your being sexy does not come from your being discovered or chosen by someone else. Instead, sexiness comes from being comfortable enough with yourself so that you become available to explore the depths of others. Your sexiness becomes a stew of calm, positive self-regard, your sensual awareness, and your interest in others.

What can you as a woman do about rape? A lot of you women have learned self-defense, and you carry Mace. You look over your shoulder a lot and are much more careful whose car or apartment you enter. That's good, though you're still working on a symptom and not the disease. I've taught college-level human sexuality classes and, thinking back, I talked about the seeds of rape when I covered dating and seduction. How many movies and romance novels have the hero moving in for a sweaty embrace with a perpetually virginal young thing who says "yes" with her eyes, "no" with her lips, until she stops pounding on his well-developed back and swoons into sexual submission? What's the message? That women don't make up their own minds about having sex. They have to be seduced, taken, coerced against their resistance. That's called passionate romance. Perhaps women have contributed to the creation of this atmosphere of associating great sex with the overcoming of their resistance by not taking frank responsibility for being sexual.

What does being liberated mean? There's a new book out for men, extolling the virtues of the new, nonmacho, sensitive, sharing, caring man. Fine. But in this book, the author warns about those women who say and think they are liberated, but still want it both ways. They want respect but still want to be treated like princesses. The author hints that these women will undermine your search to be the perfect liberated male. Wait a minute. What does "liberated" mean? "Nonliberated" refers to people caught in role traps. Does "liberated" simply mean that we're to be in new role traps? "Liberated" means freed from imposed structure with the opportunity of finding a lifestyle that makes you comfortable. And for many of you, giving up all the more traditional aspects of behavior, thought, and expectation is not what makes you the most comfortable or happy. Being Liberated is being free to choose from everything—not just so-called new ideas.

What is flirting really for? I was being interviewed the other day to make an appearance on a new cable program on sexuality. They decided not to use me because I couldn't come up to the raunchy standards they had set, but something interesting came out of it anyway. The topic was to be flirting. The flirting of yesteryear was us women types looking seductive but embarrassed, promising but innocent, and denying it all if asked directly. I suggested that the best kind of flirting for women today was simply to be direct, talkative, interesting, and interested. The interviewer said, "But what if the guy is all freaked out and turned off by that direct approach?" For a moment, I was flabbergasted. It seemed to me that she was expressing a rather ancient notion that women were to attract any man, not look around for one that was interesting and worthy enough for us. If anyone freaks out at the frank and honest version of you, what use are they to you anyway?

Drinking isn't funny or sexy. There are commercials that show how to shake it loose after a hard day's work with a drinking bash at a local bar. Others show people motivated to excel in sports by the promise of a beer. Still others equate sexual seduction and friendship with drinking. Comics often use the verbal ramblings and physical incoordination of a drunk as a source of humor. In counseling people, I haven't seen the fun, sexy side of drinking. I've seen child and spouse abuse, job losses, talent dissipation, alienation, severe illness, sexual problems, and vehicular murder. And few of those people would admit to abusing alcohol. Except for one man who finally got scared. He called me last Christmas Eve. He'd been out of town for one day to an important business meeting. He was calling me the next morning from a phone booth. He'd woken up still out of town in his car reeking from drinks. For the first time, he'd blacked out. What will it take for you?

Do you want your partner to be more interested in sex? Maybe you've read some articles, had some conversations, seen some films about sex. Sex with creativity, abandon, erotic energy, fantastic passion. Now you go to your partner and try to get them involved. You tell them how they should think, feel, and behave sexually. You push for experimentation. And you can't figure out why your lover is less interested than they've ever been. Sex is a personal, intimate, sensitive issue. It's important for you to be aware that making such requests all at once might make your partner feel inadequate and disappointing to you. Surely you realize that those feelings don't make one feel sexy. Make sure that your suggestions don't sound like demands or criticisms. And if your partner needs some time to move into this new, exciting, yet maybe somewhat embarrassing way of viewing and experiencing sex, don't show impatience. Demands, criticisms, and impatience don't make you very sexy to your partner, you know.

Hanging on to the miseries and disappointments of your past? Sometimes the fights you get into with your beloved are scattered, without focus, without point. That makes it very hard to resolve anything. Hurt and angry feelings get stuffed back into an already overfilled suitcase of resentment, and it doesn't take much for the fastenings to snap, dumping old and new material for the next fight. I doubt this is making you happy. It probably leaves you feeling at odds with your beloved, and that does little to maintain inner peace, communication, sexual attraction, and pleasure. So what could be so important to you that you'd sacrifice all of that and more to stay in this pattern? Keeping score, keeping even; making sure that you are never one down, defeated, controlled, or dominated. And boy, do you ever stretch reality to fit it into that fearful mold. Check out your fears about needing someone, about not being in control, about not trusting love.

Why are you so negative? Are you always imagining the worst is going to happen? Are you always pointing out all the ways things can and often do go wrong? Are you always ready with "aha" when things turn out crummy? I'm sure that those instances of being right don't really make you feel all that triumphant and happy inside. Before everyone labels you a curmudgeon, a scrooge, a doomsayer, let's look at what's really going on. Being negative is a means of self-protection. It's related to the "Don't get too excited and you won't get too disappointed" school of thought. Negativity is a protection against disappointment. It's also a replacement for hoping. In life, hoping is often disappointment postponed. Some so-called negativity might be useful if it keeps you thinking of all the alternatives, good or bad, so that you'll be sharp with contingency plans. One hundred percent optimism or pessimism is unrealistic and unsatisfying. A balance of childlike wishfulness and adultlike caution could be a powerful blend.

You're in a long-term affair with a married man and you don't know what you should do. Generally, the letters from women going with married men have some elements in common. "He's wonderful." "I'm in love." "It's just this little thing about having no specific future." The last such letter I got asked for advice because she could only see her own view. What is that view? That she could never have as much as she gave? That she had to be alone on holidays, important times, times of need? That she be someone recreational instead of committal? That love always be at drive's length? What kind of view is that? It's the view of someone just like you who has dearly learned to tolerate too many losses, accept less than you need, and hang on desperately to not losing even that. It's the desperate hanging on that leads to exaggeration of someone else's worth and tolerance of their slights. Is this the day when you decide that it stops being enough?

Are you a woman who enjoys sex, but feels that something is missing? Many of you women enjoy the caressing, the kissing, the holding, and the intimacy that are the lovely part of the sexual experience. You may feel somewhat disappointed in not being able to experience an orgasm as your partner does. What should you do? First, reassure yourself with a checkup that there is nothing physically wrong. The next step is to determine which of the most usual of reasons seem to apply. The most common immediate cause of this inhibition of orgasm is self-consciousness. That's when you keep watching and waiting for yourself to function, instead of allowing yourself to be caught up in the feelings. Next comes insufficient stimulation, which may require some education and practice. After that, many of you tend to have a very careful, controlled personality style, and the letting go that enjoying sex requires is uncomfortable for you. Or it may be that sex makes you feel guilty. Think about these.

Are you stamping your foot, demanding that your partner feel sexy about you? So many people I counsel begin by saying that they have no idea why their partner won't have sex with them. They say they would never say "no." They're willing to try even kinky things. They would accommodate in every sexual way possible, yet the partner just can't seem to muster the interest. I believe it's true that they would be so totally sexually available to their partner. It may just be that what their partner needs to be sexual has nothing to do with sex. Your partner may be turned off because outside of sex you are critical. You don't do things together very often, or your demeanor is too often surly, pouty, or unhappy. The atmosphere for sex isn't all wine, candles, and music. It's emotional. Feeling close most likely leads to being closer sexually. It may just be that the first line of inquiry if you're having such a sexual problem is not a sex manual, but one on friendship.

So you're not having enough sex? As a therapist, I hear lots of people complain that they aren't having enough sex with their partners. One of the things I've noticed lately is that these people aren't doing much to earn it. Are *you?* How do you earn getting sexual attention from your partner? How about giving them some attention, sexual and otherwise? How about reconsidering your general attitude and treatment of your partner? It could be that you're blaming your partner for the lack of sexual interaction, expecting them to come on to a distracted, annoyed, tired, busy, and nonfun person that you've allowed yourself to become. Getting sex isn't your due. It's a shared experience that generally requires some buildup. No, I don't mean just foreplay, unless foreplay includes consideration, thoughtfulness, time, togetherness, sharing, and involvement. I'm talking about a real investment of your time and emotional energy. That's how you earn love and sex.

Are feeling, thinking, and behaving sexy just a distant memory to you? Remember when you felt amorous at the mere sight, touch, or whiff of your dearly beloved? Ah, nostalgia. What's happened to all that excitement? Your first tendency may be to blame your partner for not doing appealing or sexually aggressive things. Perhaps there's some truth in that. But look inside yourself first. Are you taking care of yourself the way you did, the way you should? Do you treat yourself as a man or as a woman? Do you respond to the manliness or the womanliness of your partner? In other words, do you think of yourself as other than a worker, a parent, a homeowner, a bill payer, a neighbor, or a relative? I'll bet the answer is "nope." There's an all-too-natural path for responsible, hardworking people, but the price to pay is too great: no fun, chuckles, and warmies. That's an existence which can lead to affairs, alcoholism, emotional, marital, and family problems, and physical illness. Take the time right now to approach yourself and your beloved as the warm, sensitive, sensual creatures you are yearning to be.

# CHAPTER 11

# *Perfectionism*

Being right doesn't make people love you the way you thought it would, does it? Somewhere along the line, you got the notion that for you to be loved, you had to do things right. No, more than that: perfectly. Maybe when you were a child, your family gave you attention, affection, and applause for your performance rather than for your existence. If you recognize that as your history, you may be using it against yourself now. If you see yourself threatened by the loss of love because you may not be right in some situation, clearly you're going to fight to be right. Here's the paradox. The very people you fight are the people you need love from. Fighting them so that you can win, and thereby ensure love from them, means that they have to lose the fight. Their losses don't make them feel loving toward you, the victor. Instead of showing you love, they show you resentment, and you're confused and frightened. Do you want to be loved? Stop tap dancing. Stop arm wrestling, and you start loving.

Are you always on guard? It is often advisable to be
cautious and deliberate about divulging personal information, showing your inner feelings, or even believing what others tell you, especially when they say,
"Trust me." This is the real world of ulterior motives,
manipulations, jockeying for position, double-crosses,
and taking care of number one. Sound cynical? Be
aware of the difference between acceptance of reality
and cynicism. A cynic anticipates this behavior in all
persons at all times. An accepter of reality is someone
who is aware, hence, carefully selective. A dear friend
of mine said that if anybody in the world should be
cynical and avoidant, 'tis he, for all the betrayals and
heartaches he's experienced. He's not, though. Why
not? Because he chooses to live his life maximizing
his potential for peace and enjoyment. He relishes his
friends and is clever with those others. It's too easy to
allow those pains in the neck to become the outline of
your life. Instead of preparing for battle each day, hug
someone soft.

You probably need a win. Feel a lot like you're losing
lately? Dreams not coming true? The economy put a
too-low limit to the high yield of your efforts? These

are the inescapable realities of life. It's easy to feel that life is picking on you. Actually, life doesn't pick on or pick up. Life is the milieu in which all of us struggle, survive, and sustain. Life can't be blamed for your defeats, life can't be acclaimed for your successes. Life isn't invested in doing either for you. You all need wins, and a win feels the same no matter how it's gotten. A friend of mine made it down a ski slope without breaking a bone. Even after a one-year layoff, he felt triumphant. Another friend of mine taught himself how to garden, a distraction from his disappointments in life. His blooms were breathtaking this spring. He experienced an elation he could hardly believe. Do something within your power. Create a win for yourself. Create your own win.

Why is it you always seem to need more? I remember one *Star Trek* episode where the crew of the star ship *Enterprise* was trapped on a planet where everything was provided for them. The aliens couldn't imagine the earth people wanting to leave with their every need provided for without effort. Captain Kirk explained that humans need challenge to survive. Does that mean you can never be satisfied with a job, a marriage, a family, or a friendship simply because it exists securely? Some of you behave as though that were true, as though the value of things were in the getting, not the having. Perhaps you say the challenge is so much more exciting than the ongoing experience. Perhaps you don't recognize a true challenge when you see it. Sustaining something, making it grow and expand, is a more difficult challenge than medieval conquest. You do need some challenge in your life. Challenge brings excitement and newness. You do need security in your life. Security brings safety and comfort. Don't destroy your security for the sake of excitement. Find ways to express yourself creatively, physically, mentally, spiritually, and have both.

What's so good about humility? Can you say, "Damn, I'm good," and feel comfortable about it? Do you feel like you have to underplay your intelligence or abilities in order to make or keep friends? Talking openly about your marvelous capabilities often makes people flinch. You might be called a braggart, conceited, arrogant, even when you aren't exaggerating a whit. If you underplay your accomplishments, people tell you you're fishing for compliments, or they say they admire your humility. One philosopher said that humility was excellence bowing to mediocrity. Another calls it a demonstration of true greatness. It's so confusing. When you talk about yourself negatively, you get argued with, supported. When you talk about yourself positively, you get argued with, criticized. Feeling great about yourself becomes a problem to others. If you're not being directly insensitive, if you don't have the intent to demean or embarrass, I think it would be great if you all would fess up to your greatness and support and rejoice in the greatness of others.

Are you desperate for success or love, but don't dare to try for them lest you fail? So many times, you yearn to take risks, like a love relationship, new business, back to school, a sport, but you think thrice about how bad you'd feel, how embarrassed you'd be if you didn't hit gold the first time. You look at successful people as though they were a species immune to failure and mistakes. I'm reminded of a Jules Feiffer cartoon. A man meets a guru on the road and asks, "Which way is success?" The silent guru points off to the distance, and off skips the man to reap success. Suddenly, there comes a frightening *splat,* and the man limps back bleeding and lame. "You told me success was that way. I went that way and got splatted. Guru, which way is success?" The guru silently points again into the distance, and the man goes off again, and then *splat!* The man crawls back—this time, exhausted and beaten. "Guru, I've tried that way twice. Which way is success?" Finally, the guru speaks: "Success is that way. It's just a little past *splat.*"

What can you do when you're in an impossible situation? You've been in that place. You're damned if you do and more damned if you don't. There's no pleasing everybody. Maybe there's no pleasing anybody. A good way to go is to take yourself out of the middle. You can do that by considering each option as if it existed alone. Sometimes reality and practicality become clearer when you're not comparing. Another issue is to take the total weight of this problem off your shoulders. Actually go to the principals involved in your predicament. Clarify the problems, the feelings, and ask for their input, their help. They are less likely to act like either the rock or the hard place when they get a Florence Nightingale invitation. An impossible place is usually made so by your anxiety about the unknown—what everyone else will think, feel, do, or say. The impossible becomes possible when you assess clearly your needs and feelings and recruit the rock and the hard place to help you.

What can you do about a hopeless situation which you don't want to get out of? As a therapist, I'm often asked how you can cope with a situation you cannot tolerate and will not get yourself out of. At first it seems impossible. This is my prescription: Part of not wanting to get out of this intolerable, hopeless situation may be that certain practical losses would have to be realized. To some extent, I guess I can't argue with practicality. On the other hand, what price are you putting on your peace of mind, your emotional and even physical welfare? No matter what the people or the situation are providing in terms of punishment and pain, part of your staying in the predicament is your unwillingness to give up hoping and expecting. In general, this positive thinking is fine. In some situations, it is postponing and repeating disappointment and pain. Determined to stay put? Then accept the realities of what is being offered you and seek your dreams, needs, and hopes in more responsive places.

Okay, here's the magical key to making things get easier. You asked me how working through painful feelings, difficult relationship issues, or algebra can get easier. Well, it depends. Do you want an answer which will have the job done by someone else, in your sleep, without struggle and discomfort? I don't have the answer for that. Actually, the only way you can make things get easier is by doing them enough times for several things to happen. For one, as you get more familiar with whatever it is, your anxiety about the unknown diminishes. As you try something over and over again, it gets to be second nature. Your conscious mind doesn't have to torture through each and every detail anymore. As you experience it many times, you find yourself seeing it in new ways, able to build upon it, change it. Change your attitude toward it. If it happens spontaneously, or someone does it for you—and those are both impossible anyway—you could lose the joy of conquest and the control over your own destiny. So next time, just grit your teeth and try it.

Does everyone think you are a tower of strength? "I can take care of myself" in the same breath as "Everyone thinks I'm so strong and independent. I don't know why they think that. I've got my insecurities too." This sound like you? Somewhere early in your life you got the message that if you didn't take care of yourself, no one else would. Or that giving yourself over to someone else's ministration was dangerous to mind or soul. Today, you're still protecting yourself as though all the people you've met along the way are as dangerous as those who early on taught you those lessons. It may give you pride, solace, or a sense of safety to work on looking perfectly invulnerable and self-sufficient, but it usually backfires. When you need help, no one knows it, believes it, or knows what to do about it. It's just a mystery to everyone. And when you meet and develop relationships, you work mostly on presenting an image and getting the appropriate feedback. Once the person is in your life, you find time and again that they aren't truly what you need.

Are you a human Pac Man? Like the Pac Man computer game, do you race around chewing people up, stopping momentarily only because you've gotten zapped? Are you a bottom-liner, be it profit or rules? Do you see the human element of emotions and feelings as an impediment to efficiency and pragmatism? Don't worry, I'm not going to argue with you about this. Anyway, it's probably brought you great business success or power or something, because I don't think you'd go on with something that didn't benefit you in some way. You probably live and handle yourself in the way you feel the most competent, with the tools you're most familiar with, and that's what saddens me for you. I regret that you've grown up to fear emotions and vulnerability, that you're not more comfortable with gray areas, secret successes, touching experiences. You act like a computer today because there is a mercenary need for your talents—the talents which are your protection against the pain of feelings and intimate interactions. Remember, it's always possible to change the program.

Now why can't you be perfect? You strive to be perfect—in general, or just at something. You get all sick and nervous because no matter how hard you try, you're just not perfect. I've looked around for perfection. My eyebrows, pre- or postplucking, never really match each other. No matter how much I tend to my house plants, some of the leaves just dangle there limply. No matter how much I prepare and plan, something goes awry. If I practice something a hundred times, it still may not come out right the next time. What is perfection, and what's so good about it anyway? Fried chicken is perfect to me when it's cold. Is that how it's perfect to you? No? Then perfection doesn't have just one form? Now I'm confused. If I can't pin down perfection, how can I become perfect? I've had moments of perfection. Like the time I hit that backhand three millimeters over the net, right into the corner of the tennis court. The other player sailed it right back for a winner, so perfection doesn't necessarily even mean you're always going to win. So how about doing things the best way you can do at the time, in a way that gives you pleasure?

Do you put time into worrying about how smart or how good you are at things? Do you worry if your age, your gender, your situation, your background, or whatever might work against you? Worrying like this is the same as lowering your feet into drying cement. It will keep you from going anywhere, much less to the limit of your potential. I'll bet you are your own worst critic. This gives you the power and responsibility, I think, to be your own best fan, too. Worry and comparisons are not motivators. As a steady diet, they are immobilizers. If you worry enough about how good you are, you won't have the time to test yourself to find out how good you could become. Remember that word "become." Worries and comparisons are either observations or distortions of only one point in time. Unfair, irrelevant. You are always becoming. A metamorphosis. Enjoy the process of becoming, being, growing, learning, living.

Could your physical pain be a lifesaver? One lady I know was never happy or satisfied with anything she did or experienced. It should have been more. It should have been better. She could never allow herself to take time off, rest, play, or enjoy anything. Just work. She finally came to understand that the only way she could give herself permission to stop was to have a terrible headache. Her headache pain saved her from seeing herself as lazy. Her pain was real. Your pains are real, too, and they do hurt. If you're having trouble getting rid of your pain, maybe even wanting to, it may be that it protects you from something you feel is worse. Pain is relative. It is more painful for you to confront authority, risk rejections, be vulnerable with your creativity, show independence and initiative. Next to those, a perpetual headache might seem like a blessing. Check with your physician. Take the time to think about how your pain might be a way you cope.

People who charge through life are often admired for their energy and guts. Maybe in some ways they're as successful as the light brigade. In a recent exposé on drugs and sports, a famous, now retired basketball star talked about why he never used drugs. He said that he wanted to experience life at its own pace. I was struck by the profound simplicity of that statement: "Experience life at its own pace." So much of your life might be filled with racing life's pace and then paying for it later. Like when you drink to unwind and reduce the stress. Or when you have to heal your bones or mourn someone's death because you were speeding in your car. Or when you pushed intimacy to appear, and then had to deal with hurt feelings or an untimely pregnancy. It's important for you to realize things take time, and you have to give things the time they take. You have to do that without hating yourself for not being a magician or a god. If you see life as a series of end points to be rushed at, then you see cupcakes to be gulped whole, rather than savored.

What can you do about things you can't do anything about? There are lots of things you can do with things you can't do anything about. You can yell and scream or threaten or pout. You could make yourself sick with upset and worry. You could become sad and demoralized. You could give up in the hope that the universe will be so upset by your giving up that the laws of physics will be changed to accommodate you. Or you could find something over which you have some control and start building up your mood, security, and fulfillment all over again. Most of all that other stuff is your childlike wishfulness, hoping that some kind of resistance on your part has the power to change the inevitable. For your own sake, you must learn to accept what you cannot change without paying a deep psychological price as though it were your fault, thinking you failed or were inadequate. I'm not talking about giving up or giving in. But when you can't help things, help yourself.

"You can pretend anything and master it." That quote is from Milton Erickson, a master hypnotherapist. I read it to a person I'm working with in therapy and he countered with, "So what? Pretending isn't real." Isn't it?" I was taking tennis lessons from a seventy-five-year-old ex–tennis pro who could barely walk across the court. He didn't have to. He could place that ball on a dime so that I had to run all over the court. Too often, I'd get all frustrated trying to get a shot right by doing it over and over and over again until I wanted to scream. My teacher called me over and asked me to stop trying so hard. He told me to pretend. Pretend I was, say, Billie Jean King, making that perfect stroke. Back out on the court, I waited, imagining myself hitting the ball just like Billie Jean King. And before I was aware of it, I made that shot effortlessly. No, pretending isn't real, but it just might give you the opportunity to see what you can really do.

Are you good at letting someone else have the fun of being right? You know how great it feels when you're right? For that moment, you feel wonderful, lovable, fun-filled, superior, and generally terrific. Well, when you're wrong, do you make sure you contribute to the other person's experiencing all those great feelings? Or when it's proven you're wrong, do you just give in? Worse yet, do you just ignore the whole thing, hoping it will go unnoticed? Come on, you'll feel less crummy about being wrong if you expend positive effort to let the other person have some fun with being right. Instead of wallowing in embarrassment or building up resentment against your friend or beloved, say right to them, "You know, you're right. I should have bet against myself and won some money on this. Maybe I'll think of that next time." You'll survive the disappointment in yourself better, and the relationship will be less bruised by any potentially vengeful feelings of being one down if you just help someone else celebrate being right.

Why can't you walk away from a fight? You may avoid walking away from potential as well as already initiated battles. Maybe it's because you don't want to look weak or frightened. It might be with weapons, fists, or vocal cords. No matter which, you go for blood to make a point. Remember the old cowboy movies? Whenever someone didn't want to fight, he was called yellow, a baby, or a girl. Faced with these alternatives, he was usually motivated to battle and rarely won. The ethic portrayed was that it was better to be dead than to walk away from a confrontation. This mentality always imposes a value judgment imposed on you by onlookers, usually voyeuristic, gutless wonders. Don't let your sense of courage be decided by others, no matter how dirty their threats and name-calling. The greatest courage is to maintain your own sense of self in the face of the challenge of others. Remember the old *Kung Fu* series? Kane intimidated his opponents with his willingness to be challenged and maintain inner peace. That's the real triumph.

Are you sure what you're doing is procrastination? I think it's important to know whether what you sometimes do is procrastination or not. Procrastination is generally guilt-provoking, and that can ruin your whole day. Sometimes you've set aside some time to do something, and being a good scout, you sit yourself down and turn on the switch but nothing happens. You're not a vacuum cleaner. It is possible that the time you spend forcing yourself to stay in that chair is wasteful and demoralizing. That time might be better spent in some other endeavor. Maybe funsies. Maybe no. If you're always trying to avoid the noxious label of procrastinator by forcing yourself into moments of creativity or enterprise when your psyche isn't ready, you will experience enough failures and frustrations to turn yourself off completely. Trust yourself, test yourself. Give yourself time frames rather than starting guns. Give yourself rewards for jobs well done. Give yourself permission to miss a few. You might find yourself more enthusiastic about your tasks.

How can you better cope with a situation you can't stand but have to stay in? Whether it be for finances, favors, or fears, there are times it seems better to stay in a situation that's driving you crazy than leave. Yet every day you literally go crazy trying to accept the unacceptable. Impossible? No. Indeed, there are times you have to be practical. Here's how to cope. First, accept that you are doing it for, as an example, the income. Really accept that reality. Second, make that your only expectation. Once you do that, annoyances will be easier to cope with because you don't expect anything but that weekly paycheck. Third, once you get yourself into that mode, it will be easier to play with the situation. Find a way to make it amusing. No matter how bad it is, there is always something you can squeeze out of it to appreciate. As you can see, the main object of coping with horribly difficult situations is to construct a way of looking at it as though it were on your terms.

Are you just all pooped out? One woman I counsel was a terrific hairdresser. She worked professionally at two shops. She came to me with a decision to make: which job to give up because she felt so exhausted. But when we examined the two workplaces thinking about part-time shifts and such, it became clear that those jobs gave more to her than they took away. Looking deeper into her life, we realized that she gave away much of her spare time by giving free haircuts to friends and those sent by friends. Now those jobs took more than they gave. Not able to say no? Spending all of your time giving stuff away? It's likely that you are giving so much in order to get liked, to avoid others' anger or disappointment. What enslaves and exhausts you is the never-ending requirement to build and maintain your identity and worth on only that foundation. How about a foundation of self-acceptance?

Oh, come on, what's all this stuff about not having the time? You don't have the time to walk your dog, your child, or your beloved? You don't have the time to ride a bike or take a hike? You don't have the time to take a class or run out for a pass? How about seeing some sights or climbing some philosophical heights? What *do* you have time for? I know what you're going to tell me. You have lots of responsibilities you have to take care of. All sorts of people are counting on you. Take some notice. How many of those closest to you, including yourself, are benefiting from your overwhelming sense of responsibility? You're a hero out there and a figment of imagination closer to home. That sounds like a life geared for image, ego, and identity, rather than the texture of experience, warmth, and being. It's not that you don't have the time, it's that it's all spent trying to synthesize a you. Perhaps you're so busy trying, you haven't noticed that there's always been a you to express.

Indulge yourself! Responsible, hardworking people like you deserve to indulge themselves more often than you do. Do you feel guilty indulging yourself? Naughty? Childish? Those are all feelings you force upon yourself in your usual "good person" routine to keep yourself being a responsible, hardworking giver. Like any other equipment, this routine sometimes gets stuck in the giving mode, and like any other machine which isn't gassed, oiled, and generally maintained, it begins to run down and break down. In human terms, you call it burnout. That's when you become exhausted, cynical, disgusted, angry, testy, and just spent. When you're stuck in the giving and doing mode, your yield generally drops way out of proportion to your effort. What you used to see as minor rewards or interesting challenges become major and boring irritations. Want to protect the quality of your giving? Indulge yourself. When you feel filled and cheerful, you are more willing and able to give and to do.

Are you having trouble trying to come up with sufficient motivation to make a very difficult change in your life? Change is naturally difficult. It substitutes the unknown for the familiar. Discomfort, even fear, is normal. If you find yourself feeling stuck, depressed, and angrily saying that you just can't seem to find any good reason to change things, then this is you putting your own feelings and needs second, maybe even third or fifth to your disappointed rage about the past. Your own feelings are that you are simply unhappy with the way things are going. Those feelings deserve respect and attention. Why don't you provide that? Perhaps because in the past, people, maybe your family, didn't treat you in the way I'm suggesting you treat yourself now, with loving respect. It's a mistake that they didn't treat you better then. It's a mistake if you don't treat yourself better now. Indeed, if you do, you will inspire new people to do the very same.

Sometimes it is the principle of the thing. The father on *Little House on the Prairie* was confused by his wife's giving permission for him to do something she had been terribly furious and upset about, simply because he said he wouldn't do it if it upset her so much. His wife said, "Now that I know you were willing to give it up for me, I don't mind your doing it." The point was, and often is, that it wasn't the thing that had top priority in her guts. It was the feeling that he cared enough about her to give up something for her. With that awareness, she was willing to use her strength to survive the ordeal of letting him go fulfill his dream. So many times you and your beloved argue the thing and won't give in to each other's emotional needs and feelings. That's sad, because therein lies the power and the beauty of a good relationship, and the solving of what seemed impossible problems. Next time you two are arguing over something, change gears and share with each other the underlying feelings. I'll bet you'll find a solution.

What's the best way to negotiate? If to you, negotiation means getting everything you want the way you want it, you probably will never succeed. Negotiation is a fine art of ending up with both parties feeling that the other gave in or gave up on enough significant points for each to feel comfortable with their compromises. When you give the gift of giving up some part of what you want, you show the others that their feelings and needs count. This will make them more comfortable and positive about you. If it means everything to you to maintain a rigid stance, not to compromise, not to give an inch, remember, the price will be that you will get back the same or worse in return. So be practical. Decide what it is that really matters—excessive pride or the successful resolution of a troublesome situation. Once you decide what's most important to you, realize that your negotiating partner has priorities and feelings, too.

"If I have ten things to do, I cannot relax until all ten are done. Nine aren't enough." Does that sound like you? Then you have been robbed of your power to make choices. If you feel that you have to take care of that one last thing before you can go on to other things, then you have given your personal power over to some little voice which says, "You can't hug your lover. You can't giggle with your child. You can't enjoy a warm tub, read anything interesting, or do anything at all until everything is perfect." What that voice is really saying is, "You don't deserve happiness, pleasure, or choices." It's saying, "You must earn them by being perfect," which is impossible. I don't care how

hard you try. It's time to squelch that voice and re-
place it with your own freedom to smell the roses. If
anything can be perfect, that's it.

Do you know how to apologize? If it's uncomfortable
for you to admit to error or obnoxiousness, you'll
probably get defensive and just make it worse.
Demanding immediate forgiveness after your cursory
apology is your attempt to make the injured party
look like the bad guy. That's when you say, "Look, I
apologized, what more do you want? Why can't you
just let it go?" Another defensive ploy of yours to
avoid the discomfort of apologizing is to make the victim feel responsible. "Well, I wouldn't have had to get
so angry if you hadn't given me that look." Now, come
on. Is that really all it takes to get you into a mean
mode? Do you try to make believe it all just didn't
happen? Do you try to act sick and hurt to distract
your victim his their pain? Do you maintain an angry
pose for the intimidation value? All of these defensive
ploys are used by you to win, look strong, and appear
right. None of these defensive ploys gets you loved.
Sorry about that!

Are you postponing your life? Some of you live totally in today, allowing the moment's whim and impulse to design your existence. There are those of you who dream of such things as letting go, making changes, taking chances, or just being more easygoing about things. It seems intriguing . . . well, maybe someday. And so it goes that you postpone your life till maybe never. I know you are a responsible, functioning person. Don't lose that! A life regulated by choice is far better than a life regulated by fear. Choice is expanding; fear is constricting. Routines, for example, help you plan, get things done, and feel secure. That's good. Not being able to deviate from routine without experiencing immobilizing discomfort is not good. This kind of rigid adherence to the familiar is your attempt to always do the right thing and be a good little boy or a good little girl. In the immortal words of Ralph Edwards, "This is your life." Use it well.